I0134808

This book is for you if...

- You suffer from mental ill health, need to find the inner courage to open-up and want those around you to have a deeper understanding of your suffering.

- You want to help a friend, acquaintance, work colleague or loved one to come to terms with their situation.

- You are passionate about protecting the mental health of your children, grandchildren, or even your unborn children, and the generations to follow.

- You are advancing in your educational journey and want to give yourself a great advantage in the adventure of life, then the knowledge contained in this book, relating to our collective mental health and how you put it to good use, will prove to be priceless.

This Book Will Help You If...

- You recognise the mental health crisis encircling us in the modern world. A crisis fuelled by the thinly veiled and wholly unjustifiable embarrassment, shame and disgrace surrounding this serious health issue. The flaming inferno which this crisis represents, is being fanned by a wholesale lack of funding which – completing the vicious circle – has been justified by the unchecked attitude we have all had towards our mental health. Until now.

- You want to play your part in dismantling the so-called stigma surrounding mental health. This book will give you the gift of knowledge and tools to spread its message throughout the world. The core belief of the community which blossoms from the seeds sown by this book will make the required funding available to mark the beginning of the end of the global mental health crisis.

About the Author

Tony Weekes grew up in East London, the son of a consultant surgeon and a nurse. Following his education to degree level, he worked his way up to office management level. The combination of his upbringing, life and work experience has made him see the good in every situation and solve any problem that confronts him as it arises.

He has witnessed the pain and suffering, which mental ill health has caused several of his extended family members, and at times has found this overwhelming. As a result for the past few years he has devoted all of his energy, enthusiasm and determination into generating solutions for the problems they faced.

Tony has built and coordinated the Unity Team. Unity is his vision of how the stigma of the United Kingdom's (UK) mental health problems can be dismantled; how effective ongoing treatment can be made accessible; and how socio-economic empowerment for sufferers can be provided as the result. Tony has built this caring community – not from the perspective of a professional in the field of mental health - but from first hand experience of trying to ease the suffering of his loved ones. He has tried, sometimes succeeded, other times failed, to surmount the problems caused by the current care system's serious lack of funding and the resulting lack of cohesion.

He says the biggest lesson he has learnt is the role of the family in securing treatment for someone suffering mental ill health is second only to the acknowledgement of the person suffering.

Unity is a grassroots movement to revolutionise mental health care in the United Kingdom through education, recognition and intervention. The UK's National Health Service (NHS) is a world leader in health care and Tony wants to establish Unity as a leader in mental health care. His vision, shared in this, his first book, is of Unity Mental Health Service – Unity MHS - becoming world renowned and helping people right across the globe.

What Other People Are Saying About This Book

"This is a well-presented book about mental health in the UK today, which will help to raise awareness of the sheer scale of the problem, particularly among younger people. For a long time I have harboured concerns about the stresses that youngsters face today and the effect on their wellbeing. This book not only raises awareness of this but also points to contributing factors that may not at first seem obvious.

This book is certainly thought-provoking. I have some personal experience of the effect of mental illness on the lives of younger people and I have not always been able to begin to understand how or why these individuals came to be affected as they were. This work indicates a number of potential causes including: addictive behavior; family and peer pressure; and diet, which all should be considered.

I recommend this book to the widest possible audience in the hope that awareness of the nature of the problem will allow more positive actions to prevent problems and for carers to understand and help those suffering."

Geoffrey E. Hawkes, BSc, PhD, FRSC, CCHem,
Professor Emeritus, Queen Mary, University of London

"This book is an eye-opener for us all. The fact that Tony is speaking from years of first-hand and heart-breaking experience, of supporting family members with mental health issues and the alarming lack of emergency and ongoing medical treatment they have endured, immediately engages the reader's interest and empathy. Tony has also researched thoroughly and quotes from reliable sources, which provides the proof that what he is saying cannot be ignored.

As you read through each chapter, you increase your awareness about the devastating and far-reaching effects that the current layers of seemingly unconnected issues we all face on a daily basis are eroding the health and wellbeing of current and future generations. The sheer number of people either suffering or affected by mental health issues is at first unbelievable. But as you read on it becomes glaringly obvious that we are in the midst of an undeniable humanitarian crisis on our doorsteps, which most of us are oblivious to!

I taught in primary education for 25 years and whole-heartedly believe that training teachers to recognise the signs of stress at the early stages and support children and young people before they become desperate and resort to addiction and self-harm, would be a huge step towards increasing career prospects and reducing the number of people who start their adult life battling alone with anxiety and depression etc.

The good news is that the ordeals Tony has encountered have spurred him on to find a workable solution. I encourage every reader to explore further the aims of Unity MHS to see how we can all make a difference and be part of the change that is crucial to society.

I acknowledge Tony for his strength and tenacity in all the hard work he has put in to help, not only his family, but all of our families. Each journey begins with one small step. I believe the publication of this book is the first step on a far reaching journey and I wish Tony every success along the way."

Linda Grandson, retired Head Teacher

"Tony Weekes writes a thoughtful and tender account of his experiences dealing with mental health issues. He writes clearly and with feeling and provides incredible insight into the challenges faced by those caring for someone with a mental health condition.

Not only does Tony write about his personal family experiences, but he also raises a number of pertinent and tough questions in an attempt to discover why mental health issues are on the rise. Are we not disciplining our children properly? Is the food we eat damaging us? Is there too much sugar in our diet? Are we genetically programmed to struggle with mental health problems at some point in our lives? These questions and many more will challenge the way we view mental health and how we can take positive steps to protect ourselves, and our families.

This is a must-read book for everyone. We will all be exposed to mental health problems at some point in our lives - whether ourselves or our loved ones - and this book goes some way to help insulate us from the complications that can arise from such issues.

Ideally this should be part of the school curriculum – in the future - so every child in the country can read and learn from it. Hopefully that will help to raise a generation who are more educated in this field and are better prepared for what life has to throw at them."

Leon Wingham, Director, Red Chilli Publishing

"I really enjoyed reading Tony's first book. It presents a fantastic mission statement and a reference of how people can gain help, even though there is still an enormous amount of stigma associated with mental illness.

His book gives us a real insight into what it is like living with someone with this illness. And I agree with him that the police need to be trained in dealing with people who have mental health conditions if they have the ability to decide if somebody should be taken into care. The current lack of long-term solutions throughout the system, leads patients back into the same situations.

I support Tony's passion and quest to encourage primary and secondary schools to include mindfulness and meditation for their pupils. As well as his case for pastoral care teachers to be trained to look out for the signs of mental health conditions in children or for schools to have a specialist trained member of staff.

I highly recommend this book to my friends, family, colleagues and clients, because it provides a tremendous insight to what mental illness is and its many forms. It also shows what we can all do collectively to help the sufferers of this affliction. I wholeheartedly agree with the points that Tony makes about: general health; food; the environment; chemicals; and how these cause such imbalances."

James Dunne, Personal Trainer, Mind Body Detox

Dedications

To my fiancée and our two children –
my inspiration – my life.

To the seven billion of us all – change our thinking –
and we can truly change the world!

Tony Weekes

Acknowledgements

There are members of my family who suffer from varying degrees of mental ill health. Unfortunately, the stigma surrounding their illness means that for their own wellbeing, I cannot divulge exactly who they are as it could possibly lead to their decline. However, they have served as the inspiration and the driving force behind the spark of an idea, which resulted in me writing this book.

Once my idea had taken the form of a miniature seed that had been firmly planted within my mind, I approached my Godmother – Linda – to ask if she knew of someone who could help me build a website. She introduced me to a lady called Vinetta. Little did I know that I had met the person who has been a pillar of strength in all aspects of everything which followed. Whenever I have encountered an obstacle which has taken me hours of pondering to plot courses around it, she has squashed any such obstacle in a single breath. Without her wisdom, I have no doubt that this organisation would be nowhere near as strong as it is right now. My unofficial equal in everything that I have officially sought to do.

My official Deputy, Simon has always challenged my every plan as much as I would expect him to. Our debates have always kept me on my toes and honest to the overall objectives.

Even though we do not always agree, the fact that we keep moving forward at a pace that suits our situation leaves me in no doubt that our partnership will continue to flourish now and in the future.

To all the followers we have amassed so far, your belief in the objectives of the organisation are driving it forward at pace and will ultimately ensure that it is a success. Thank you so very much for all your ongoing support.

To my book coach and editor, Wendy Yorke, who helped to make this book a reality and empowered my writing to go out to the world. Thank you.

Author's Message

Please join our community through the Unity website and spread the message of this book, to help people around you now and future generations.

www.unity-mhs.org/join

In my Right Mind

One man's quest to challenge our thinking on mental well-being

Tony Weekes

Founder: unity-mhs.org

Filament Publishing

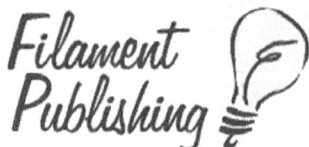

Published by
Filament Publishing Ltd
16, Croydon Road, Waddon, Croydon,
Surrey, CR0 4PA, United Kingdom
Telephone +44 (0)20 8688 2598
Fax +44 (0)20 7183 7186
info@filamentpublishing.com
www.filamentpublishing.com

ISBN 978-1-912256-29-7

Printed by IngramSpark

Contents

Introduction:
Mental Health in the UK – A Reality Check

Please take a moment and ask yourself how many families are going through the angst of mental ill health? Not only in the UK: but worldwide. With your help, this story may yet have a positive outcome. Not just for one family, but the millions of families throughout the UK and worldwide suffering with a loved one going through heartbreak.

Mental ill-health has almost torn my family apart. Two of our loved ones have suffered from long-term mental instability. It built up, along with our guilt at not recognising it sooner, to the point where their situation was spiraling towards oblivion. They were either missing, homeless and sleeping rough, or they were in temporary accommodation until they went missing again, or they ended up in hospital. They had no job prospects due to their illness, which probably made them feel worthless. And that feeling of worthlessness was probably made worse by having to exist on benefits. They were plummeting towards rock bottom.

Sustained periods of medical treatment helped, but it is short term and inconsistent, which made it ineffective and probably pushed them further towards rock bottom. The mental health system is like any family – who have been torn apart – with everyone pulling in different directions. Add to that the perceived shame and disgrace attached to mental health and it has left our loved ones alone, with nowhere to turn and a sense of being utterly lost.

This has to change and with your help it will.

Mental health is one big grey area. To overcome it, everything must be black and white.

When all the families and the friends of sufferers, along with professionals and society as a whole, take on the core belief as a unit that there is no shame or disgrace surrounding mental illness, it can be beaten. The strength that unity gives the system will allow treatment to be ongoing, consistent and effective. Over time that will allow sufferers to gain greater mental stability, a home of their own and in time, job prospects, and the ability to regain their self-worth.

Ultimately, their recovery – not just for now but for life – can be rock solid.

This can happen, through the conception of Unity as an organisation.

Join our community, through the Unity website and spread the message of this book, to help people around you now and future generations: **www.unity-mhs.org/join**

*'I do not think I suffer from mental ill
health or addiction, so I
am all good! But… by their very nature,
that may mean that I do!'*

Tony Weekes

PART ONE:

I

Tony Weekes

Chapter 1:
Who am I?

Somehow I'd reached the High Road. As I got to the corner by the supermarket that I frequented, childhood memories made me shiver, but they were only distant blurs in my subconscious. I didn't know what time it was, although it was dark. The air was filled with a fine mist and a serene calm, although I was the only person there; accompanied only by a deep-seated sense of fear somewhere within me. Suddenly, I noticed two of the young lads I used to work with crossing my old road and heading towards the rear of the supermarket. Walking towards them, I tried to get their attention but they didn't hear me even though they were only a short distance away.

'Strange,' I thought. 'Oh, well. They're probably up to some mischief as usual. Let them get on with it.'

I carried on along the road, which I'd been up and down so often while growing up. With each step I took, it seemed to be getting darker and the serene calm was changing into an intense silence more and more deafening. I knew where I was going and I was happy to be going there, but the fear and anticipation of what I might find grew and grew.

As I approached the drive way I saw our two dogs. Susie, the majestic character of a Labrador combined with the fearsome loyalty of an Alsatian, and Kim, a mixture of every character a dog can possess. It looked like they were trying to pull off one of their frequent escapes. Both of them seemed to notice my presence at the same time because they swiftly went back through and into the house as I got to the driveway, seemingly showing me the route I knew I had to take. Both of the front doors were wide open. The main light from the hallway shone out into the darkness like a beacon.

I paused at the entrance to the driveway, taking in - for a second - the dark magnificence of the house and the memories cocooned within. Then I thought, I must see who's in and let them know the dogs almost got out. As I took my first few steps along the driveway, it seemed as though my fear had disappeared. I got closer to seeing through the open doors and into the hallway. Suddenly, before I reached the doors, the fear came back, now with full force from nowhere, like a bullet hitting my flesh. I didn't double over though, I froze.

An imposing, mature West Indian male figure appeared in the doorway. He came out in a direction that would pass me by inches. I could not see what he was wearing in the dark night environment, but I imagined it was his well-kept leather shoes, smart trousers and one of his tweed blazers with a shirt underneath, undone at the collar. I wanted so much to scream, to laugh, to cry or to just say hello, but I couldn't. I was frozen to the spot, open-mouthed as he continued until he was almost level with me.

As he approached, I saw his face in perfect clarity - quite round with handsome and well-defined features - a reasonably short head of hair and a greying goatee. I looked into his eyes and the fear, pain and frustration at not being able to say or do anything became almost unbearable. His eyes were completely wide open, un-blinking like two full moons with brown pupils instead of craters, staring with intense force directly into mine. The intensity of the stare was virtually mind blowing, as though I had done something terrible.

The fear, pain and frustration grew so much inside me that I felt my breath getting shorter and heavier as though I was sprinting. He passed me and the intense glare continued for as far as we could both turn our necks. I think it was the sound of my breath, which woke me. I sat bolt upright in bed, recaptured my breathing and wiped the sweat from my brow. As I put my head in my hands I silently screamed inside my head – Dad!

I had that dream only days after the sudden death of my father. More than seven years have now passed and the dream lives on in my memory, as though I had it just yesterday. I have always felt – rightly or wrongly – that the intensity of the glare represented some form of anger. But anger at what, me? At what had mysteriously happened in the time immediately before and after he passed away? Or anger at what was to come? I'm not sure whether I believe that his soul could foresee what was to come but I have asked myself anyway. Could it be the failure of the business he left us with? My recent – now discharged - bankruptcy? The suffering which my whole family has been through during recent times while I have been at the helm? Or the struggle I have had in keeping the promise I made his soul just prior to his funeral, when we spent our last minutes alone, him lying in state? I will never know. What I do know is that I will never give up on keeping that promise. Never, ever, ever…

I have realised that in fulfilling the promise I made to my father – may he soon rest in peace if he is not already – I may in some way be able to help society at large. Help those families struggling to make ends meet for a common reason and help those on their own, who through utter desperation feel that there is absolutely no hope for them.

To my mother, I know how you have struggled to cope with the situation which surrounds us. The sometimes seemingly superhuman strength you have shown has always given me inspiration. Please be as sure as you can be that I will not stop until the changes I seek are in place and the people you know and love, who are so badly in need of care, get exactly that. Proper care. This is my promise to you.

Before I take you – the reader – on a journey that will hopefully represent our first step together on the ladder to doing exactly that, let me introduce myself.

By looking at me and my upbringing, you would think I'm a Labour man at heart – slightly left of centre and wholeheartedly on the podium for workers' rights - I am not.

Take note of my education and you would think I'm Conservative in my beliefs. Solidly on the Right – promoting competition between people and agreeing with the principle that if they reach the top through sheer hard work and effort, then they are where they deserve to be. As is everyone else. I am not.

If you were to analyse my ideals, you would believe that I am a Liberal, fighting against injustice wherever it is found through the power of speech alone. I am not.

What you will read in this book may make you feel certain I am a Revolutionary. That I am looking to change the system from top down; to install another system of power. I am not.

I am human and I am by no means perfect, that is what makes us human. I believe in humanity and in the core values of life, including, happiness, love, peace, freedom, safety, intelligence, respect, equality, justice, nature, human health and trying to learn from our mistakes. The sad fact that these core values have been almost worn down to the bone without us realising it is something we all need to comprehend as we set off on the first step we take together. All I ask of you is to set off on this journey with humanity in mind, not politics.

I do not believe in labels. In the 2015 General Election in the United Kingdom, I could not decide for love nor money who to vote for. In the end, I thought it would be easiest to vote for the party who would better my situation and made any mention of what I plan to achieve. This hardly made the decision any easier. The leader of the party I voted for resigned the next day. Great lot of good that did! If you tried to pin me down to label myself as any of the political viewpoints above, I believe in a small part of what each represents, including:

- Workers must be cared for as they generate the fuel by which the world we currently live in is driven;

- A strong work ethic, but not at the expense of others;

- Injustice must be squashed, wherever it occurs in the world, but actions speak far, far louder than words;

- That the current system of government does work. It is the master which it serves that needs to embrace humanity, not the other way around. Those in power need to have a word with themselves and remember what the core value of democracy is and who they really work for; so revolution? No. Some degree of change? Most definitely, yes.

While I was growing up – to a lesser extent – and even more so in recent times, my family has had to endure and cope with multiple episodes of mental ill health on more than one front. Throughout these times, there have been many occasions when I could have fallen off the same cliff, but I have remained strong for the sake of my family, myself, my partner and my young children. In recent times, I have witnessed second hand, how truly horrific mental illness can be and how the way it is treated is – putting it mildly – not working in any way, shape or form. I know that how this umbrella 'illness' is viewed by us and is treated by the system, desperately needs to change. I believe that once these changes happen in a certain way, the other changes that naturally follow will be a bright spark for humanity on the whole and it will be humanity who reaps the rewards in every way.

While mental health is one of, if not the most, complex issue that humanity must face up to, the plan I have devised for trying to bring about change is relatively simple. The one promise I can make you, the reader, is that with enough support, this book will bring about the required change and I will put my heart and soul into sustaining that change once it happens. Please believe, if enough people read this book, I will make these changes happen with assistance from the great people I surround myself with and driven by your support. I promise!

I was brought up to always say please and thank you. Good manners of all kinds shared between us all on a daily basis make for a brighter, nicer, happier world. And I would like to say thank you for purchasing this book. By doing so, I hope you understand that you are helping to bring about the very changes that will also make the world we live in, brighter, nicer and happier to some degree. All I ask of you is to please read what follows with an open mind, while always bearing in mind what the consequences may be for the world we return to our children, if change does not happen.

Please tell as many people you know as possible about what you have read and suggest they should also definitely read this book too.

In writing this book, I am mindful of the fact that it must be readable by anyone of the right age and maturity to be able to understand the vision I am explaining to you, the reader. In other books I have read, there is a message the writer is trying to get across or a story they are trying to tell. However, the words they use are so extravagant, long and complicated that the book is more like a work of art. I have found myself reading parts of books and knowing what they are trying to say, but having to break down the code of how they are saying it.

That is not the intention of this book, in fact, quite the opposite. My aim is for you to be able to read this book and understand it. That is why I have tried to keep the book as short as possible. Then, you can pass the vision onto your children and they can pass it on to theirs and so on. That, in the end, will help us to make sure that the intended change is sustainable.

So, if you're ready, sit down, strap in and enjoy our journey together. Hopefully, when we get to the end of the book, we can make our contribution, together, make the world a brighter, nicer and happier place.

Chapter 2:
Whose suffering serves as inspiration?

In this chapter, I will introduce you to two members of my extended family, their strengths and their weaknesses in standing up to what life throws at them, the agonising physical and mental pain they have suffered due to their illnesses, and the emotional turmoil which their suffering has inflicted on the whole family. This is a true story, which represents the inspiration that has driven my heart to demand action; now.

However, for legal reasons, specific details have been changed to protect peoples' identities, protect their psyches from the unjustifiable sense of shame which surrounds their health issues; and ultimately to protect their wellbeing.

The following quote offers a snapshot of the mountain we face.

'On most counts, young people's lives are improving. Drinking, smoking and drug-taking are down in the UK; teen pregnancies are at their lowest level for nearly half a century. Yet there is growing evidence that teens are in the grip of a mental health crisis. It is as if, rather than acting out, young people are turning in on themselves. Rates of Depression and anxiety among teenagers have increased by 70% in the past 25 years.'

Independent newspaper online (Ref. 1)

Throughout my life, there are a handful of people I know who have been through illnesses categorised as mental health conditions, of varying degrees, regardless of their age. All of them are, or have been, close to me. What separates these people is where they are in their life and the degree to which they are doing well on their life's journey; if they are still on that journey. Two of these people – two of my loved ones – have opened my eyes to such an extent that my heart is now commanding that change is needed and that change must happen.

It all started some years ago, when I was at home taking a break from work. I received a frantic phone call from one of my family, Anna. 'Get here quickly!' She begged me. 'Something terrible has happened to Stephen!'

Before I could ask what had happened, she was distracted by something or someone in the background and started screaming at them; just before hanging up. Without hesitation, I set off to find them. Although the journey was short at around 15 minutes, it seemed to take an eternity. Thoughts flew through my mind like fireworks.

I pondered my upbringing and how it had brought me to believe that family is the foundation of unconditional love, strength and support in our lives; whether it be a mother, father, sister, brother, aunt, uncle, cousin or fifth cousin. We must be there each other, regardless of any past disagreement or grievance, which must be worked through for the sake of family unity. What had Anna been screaming, as she hung up the phone? I reminded myself that in times of confrontation, Anna is always very vocal. In the same way, when she is shocked or frightened it makes her laugh out loud nervously. She will say things exactly as she sees them, while switching from her usually well-spoken manner to whatever tone, pitch and colourful language the situation dictates. I believe this is a mark not only of her intelligence and people skills, but also of how fiery her temper can be when she allows it to vent. Anna's excellence in the sporting arena – which she engages in at national level – is only matched by her incredibly competitive streak, which has driven her to win countless competitions. The importance of family and her undeterred family loyalty also flows through her veins; hence the frantic nature of the phone call. Care and compassion also run through Anna's core. When she sees someone in pain or suffering, it pains her if she cannot do anything to help. In terms of balance, I believe this is more of a strength than a weakness. All these factors really had me worried.

What had happened to Stephen? I tried not to dwell on what may have happened so I could remain focused on the rain-swept roads I was navigating. I remembered that he had been brought up with impeccable manners. And I do not know if he realises how intelligent he is. While he oozes charisma, he has always had an edge. His way with figures makes me imagine he could easily make it as a fully qualified accountant, but he has more than that. Even at a young age he has a way with the spoken word and his formulation of debate or argument could see him one day trading verbal blows with the best barristers or solicitors in the business. He is also very talented in sport, representing his county in one field and excelling locally at another. However, these traits – especially the verbal traits – can easily be viewed as arrogance or cockiness, often leading to confrontation with those at the receiving end of his occasionally misunderstood character. Could that be what's got him into some hot water?

I arrived at the scene to find that thankfully Stephen was up and standing on both feet, but there were several policemen in the vicinity – one of whom was speaking to Anna. As I got closer to Stephen, I could tell that he was very agitated, which had something to do with his face being covered in blood. I discovered that Stephen and Anna had been discussing what they should both do now that they were approaching the time they would leave school. Stephen had been giving her his heartfelt advice because it seems she was at a crossroads. One of Stephen's unmistakable features is his deep booming voice. Even when he is not talking loudly, it is almost impossible for his voice not to fill whichever room he is in. I still do not know exactly what was said or done to provoke it, if anything, but for whatever reason, Stephen was set on by a man more than twice his age and size, who had also been at the same venue for hours and had until then worked as security at a local night club.

It seemed to my untrained eye that the attack had broken his nose. Either way there was lasting damage to his nose and his ear. Little did I know the long-term effects this attack would have on Stephen. I got them both home in my car, so they could rest and recuperate with their immediate family, once I explained what had happened and the drama had calmed. Where that incident took place on the timeline of the journey that Stephen and Anna have been on since then is unclear to me now. However, in my mind that day was extremely significant.

Which came first; the chicken, or the egg?

Some months or even years before the attack, I remember learning through the family grape vine, that despite the protests of Stephen's parents and other local residents, a hostel had been allowed to open next to their family home. As I remember, its purpose was to be accommodation for ex-prison offenders. At the time of this discovery, I did not realise the significance of this development. I now understand that it was huge.

Immediately before the attack, and for a considerable period following it, the paths which Stephen and Anna were on did not conform to the initial part of the earlier quote from the *Independent*. 'Drinking, smoking and drug taking' formed a big part of both their lives. This was compounded by their increasing disconnection from their immediate families who had no real idea of the extent of their consumption. Their attitude of disconnection was put down to their natural development during their mid to late teenage years. *'It's just a phase.'*

However, the whole family were becoming increasingly concerned about Stephen. At the age of 16 he dislocated his hip playing football. This naturally meant he could not take part in any sporting activity during the long period of his recovery. This unfortunate injury coincided with his disconnection from the family.

Then came the bombshell. I remember exactly where I was on the day I heard the news because it was of such great significance and still haunts the whole family. I was sitting in my dorm at University chatting to a relative. He told me that Stephen had gone to his parents desperate for help and opening up about the trouble he was in. I heard that before the attack and over a considerable time after it, Stephen had become friends with a resident – several years older than him – in the hostel next door to his family home. It had come out that the hostel resident had been plying him and some of his friends with highly addictive class A drugs!

After that conversation, I sat and thought for a while before realising that when I first heard of the hostel, Stephen was around 16. He had been unable to play sport; his disconnection from the family. Following his admission to his family, Stephen went through a long period of rehabilitation and therapy. He got his life back on track and moved away to University. While enjoying several years of sobriety, he gained a degree in accounting and financial management from a University world-renowned in the field. He also channeled his extra energy into working out at the gym every day, building a physique which anyone would be proud to achieve. Approximately ten years after the rehabilitation, life gave him another test. Bad luck came knocking one day and he injured himself again, seriously pulling a muscle in his back. This meant no gym for several weeks, which coincided with the end of a long-term relationship. Shortly afterwards, bad luck came knocking again and the old inner demons from the hostel next door came banging the door of his mind. He answered the door and obliged.

In 2010, according to other family members - after a long period of hearing voices, hallucinations, unbelievable levels of paranoia, insomnia, starving himself to the point of losing what looked like a third of his body weight gained through all his gym work, Stephen was detained in hospital for the first time under a section of the mental health act. When the police had come across him, they were very concerned for his safety and that of the public. He was first diagnosed with Bipolar disorder, which has since been changed to Schizoaffective disorder.

In broad terms, the type of disorder which Stephen suffers from includes symptoms of schizophrenia, depression and mania. Psychiatrists believe that the causes of this illness relate to genetic, environmental and biological factors. Research cited by Rethink (a UK registered Mental Health Charity) suggests that genetically – people who suffer have a similar genetic make-up; chemically – imbalances within their brain can cause the onset of the illness; and environmentally – all aspects of their childhood, lifestyle choices and relationships can cause vulnerability to the mentally crippling illness from which Stephen suffers.

Considering these factors on the journey which he has been on since his late childhood, two out of the three forced their way into his life when he was stalked and lured in by the predator living in the hostel. The environment, which Stephen found himself in after being bitten once by the predator could have meant that the chemical balance of his brain underwent catastrophic change from that moment forwards. However, the fact that psychiatrists believe he may also have been genetically more vulnerable to this type of illness is, or should be, terrifying.

Which came first, the chicken or the egg; the addiction or the mental illness?

A leaflet produced by Mind cites research which suggests that 30-50% of people suffering from mental illness also show strong signs of alcohol and or drug misuse. While not all sufferers of mental ill health are described as having what is called a dual diagnosis, as Stephen unofficially has, many of them do. In Stephen's case, he strayed as a youngster and got back on the right track for more than a decade. Neither he, his family nor any of his friends recognised the signs of the underlying disorder, which had already taken root and he spiraled again. The complexity of his battle is that the addiction and the Schizoaffective disorder feed each other – threatening his life.

There was a period when Stephen was barely sleeping or eating at all for days on end. His mental health was plummeting towards oblivion in front of the whole family and there was nothing we could do about it. At one point, we called the Mental Health Crisis Team who told us we were powerless. All we could do if we were concerned he might do something dangerous to himself or someone else was to call the police. But we knew that, as before, the police would say there's nothing they could do because he would present as being in a reasonable condition to the officers who attended. Stephen is so articulate in dealing with other people - this is his gift - but also his curse, during an episode. We could see what the situation was building up to and we just had to watch or hear the situation unfold, while not being able to do anything about it due to the failings of the system.

During the chaos, which followed, Stephen literally went missing for weeks. We had no idea where he was from day to day. We could have reported him missing as we had in the past, but he was in contact every so often so we knew he was alive. The conversations I personally had with him were so one sided that they consisted of me trying to work out what on earth he was talking about. The code of words he mumbled seemed unbreakable, but I was met with utter verbal resentment when I could not break his code. This made me feel guilty because I thought I should be able to work out what he was talking about. Asking where he was only fuelled his paranoia, which was already at fever pitch.

When he was not in contact, the family had to wait to hear if he had called someone else or hope the call someone received was to tell us that he had been found, in one piece and had not done something absurd or dangerous. Once, we received a call from a friend saying they were very scared about what Stephen may do during what we rightly perceived to be a serious episode brought on by his illness. The friend had called the police who were on the scene.

As his closest relatives were too frail to tackle the rapidly evolving situation head-on, I took charge of the situation from our side of the family, even though I was hundreds of miles away in another part of the country. However, the police on the scene believed that Stephen and the public were not in danger. I got this information from several frantic phone calls from Stephen's friend. The police were about to leave and let him continue along his life-threatening episode because they could not see the thoughts he was having, which were fraught with danger for himself more than other people. Eventually, I spoke to the police on the phone begged the officer not to let him go – for his own safety – and to receive something resembling some help of some form. Thankfully, the police reluctantly obliged.

Although the family always felt very uncomfortable about asking the police to detain Stephen and would never usually take that course of action, we had to do this for his wellbeing. In those circumstances it is virtually the only way of knowing he is safe while in such an extremely vulnerable state. That is the dilemma, which our family have faced on the several occasions when we have been in that situation. Regardless of the uncomfortable position it puts us in, we do not regret this and will continue to do the same again and again, when necessary, on every recurrence of such an episode or crisis. The family of the sufferer is powerless in such circumstances and that solution is the only pressure release available and what pressure it is.

The hard truth is that it does not matter whether the addiction or the mental illness came first. What matters above all else, is that both illnesses are given ongoing treatment. In the same way they feed each other, surely if both are treated and are overcome to some extent, then the effects of both illnesses can diminish over enough time.

All or nothing

Anna had also been among the group of children seduced by the addictive wears distributed by the predator from the hostel. On finishing her education, she travelled to another part of the country to live with extended family while working in catering to pay her way. This seemed to be the most constructive route to take while planning what direction she wished to go in. I am unsure of the details of what happened while she lived with our extended family. However, when she returned home, Anna decided to stand up to her inner demons, which had partly been born from her contact with the residents of the hostel. They formed part of the environmental factors, along with her chemical imbalance, which led to a diagnosis of major affective disorder or severe depression and anxiety.

I remember Anna describing her type of character as being 'All or nothing'. This I think sums her attitude up perfectly. If she goes for something she will go for it 110 per cent. Along her journey so far, during the good times – following periods of various types of therapy – she will commit 110%

to a fully healthy lifestyle with absolutely no vices. Except for the occasional cigarette. Whereas, during the bad times, she will commit 110% to all the excesses, which she was first introduced to as a teenager. There is no middle ground. But what lies between the all and the nothing?

In Anna's case, I believe it is the environment surrounding her and its effect on the intricate chemical balance, which determines the all or the nothing. As noted in the quote from the *Independent*, Anna may have an ingrained habit of turning feelings inwards. As she is essentially an outgoing person, the bottling up of emotions represents the basic nature of her battle. All the pressures which life throws at Anna are either spoken about and dealt with during good times, or turned inwards during times of vulnerability, where it fuels the anxiety and depression which she suffers. This builds up to the point where she will make the split-second decision to give in to the inner demons. She will revert to going 110% in the direction of consumption, which feeds the ravenous anxiety and depression; all or nothing.

During the dark times, she has told me how she completely loses control of her emotions and seemingly sprints down a path towards physical and mental self-destruction as quickly as she possibly can. She abuses herself in almost every way imaginable, trying to relieve the inner pain she feels and her misguided perception of how those closest to her view her. The family can only look on in terror, helpless.

Thankfully, there usually comes a point when just for a few minutes, reality takes control like the sun peering briefly through the deep dark clouds in her mind. A few minutes are sometimes all it takes. Anna is strong enough in character to realise she cannot continue along her path towards self-destruction. Sometimes, after suffering for months on end, she will pause and reach out for help. However, she will normally have to wait weeks for the help that is so needed. Sometimes the pain takes hold again as the clouds drown out the sun before help arrives, so the family must remain patient while longing for another window of opportunity, a break in the clouds. On other occasions, she has the strength of will to stand up to the torture and help herself with the support of the family, until the help arrives while hoping that the mental pain she has been through has not inflicted serious damage physically.

In my opinion, Anna is one of the strongest people I have ever known through the journey she has been on. Her strength, I believe has its foundations in her mind when her 'all or nothing' attitude is positive. However, being human, her greatest weakness comes to the fore when the symptoms of depression and anxiety come boiling up to the surface and force the 'all or nothing' attitude to flip to the negative.

My standing within our family is that of the trouble-shooter or problem solver. During times of crisis for either Stephen or Anna, that responsibility places me in the eye of the storm.

Take a moment to pause and reflect on what you have just read.

Do you know someone, family or otherwise, who suffers from mental illness? When did you last see, or speak with them? How much do you think they would appreciate a call or text right now to see how they're doing?

If the above question does not apply to you, do you know anyone who has been going through an emotionally testing time recently? When did you last touch base with them to see how they're doing?

Conversations are so very good for the soul. A problem shared is a problem halved, after all.

Chapter 3:
What is my why?

If you have never witnessed a meltdown up close, then you may get a small insight from the brief outline which follows. One of the biggest insights I have gained in witnessing the plight of Stephen and Anna has been what questions need to be asked concerning poor mental health and where to find the answers.

In my opinion, witnessing someone going through an episode of mental illness is like watching from a distance as someone is walking on a very thin tightrope, trying to cross a very wide and deep canyon with no safety net. The most horrifying aspect of it is that they are extremely dizzy as they try to get to the other side. Initially, I naturally found myself asking the following questions:

- What do you think you're doing?

- What on earth are you talking about?

- What have you done to hurt yourself?

- Where have you been?

- How did you break this?

- How did you break that?

- What have you had?

- When will this end?

I reached a point when I understood that the questions I was asking were not focusing on the right area. They were material in nature. The question I, and everyone else, needed to be asking was why?

- Why would someone so intelligent do that?

- Why would someone of such inner beauty do things which are so extreme that they affect everyone around them?

- Why is he or she sleeping rough when they have a home they can live comfortably in?

- Why are they doing themselves such harm that they may end up dead as a direct result of their actions?

- Why do they not see and understand the harm they are doing to themselves and the pain they are causing to everyone around them?

By changing the approach and theoretically searching for the answers to these difficult questions, I came up with the one question which was staring me directly in the face when witnessing such extreme meltdowns. That question was: what is going on inside their tortured mind that is making their mind and body so ill?

When someone goes through mental illness, everyone around them also suffers, whether through witnessing their suffering or coping with the results of their actions or inaction. However, those around the sufferer have varying degrees of resilience, which helps them to cope.

The human brain is one of, if not the most, complex and advanced computers in the world. It is amazing to think that we may only use 10% of our brain in everything we do. There are no two people in the world who are identical; physically or mentally. It is a fact of life that we are all different, stronger in some groups of muscles for one person and other groups of muscles in another person. In the same way, I believe one person may be mentally stronger in one way than another and vice versa. We all possess varying degrees of resilience. The one point at which we are all very similar is before we are born, growing inside the womb. We are all from the same template and are born with a brain made up in virtually the same way with the same pathways.

I believe it may be our development either before we are born or when we are growing up – as in the case of Stephen and Anna – which sets the foundations for how resilient we can be and how well we can cope with the stresses and strains which modern life puts us under.

While formulating my plan to establish Unity, I had a conversation with a colleague. It was she who likened the brain to a computer and we spoke about resilience. She said that if we look at the brain as a computer, what if it is the wiring of that computer being ever so slightly faulty which can lead someone down the path towards mental illness. Taking this possible factor into consideration, I believe the wiring problem starts either before we are born or when we are growing up and throughout our childhood. Either way, I believe everyone needs to look at what we as a race of human beings are doing, which could be making this a possibility.

Ironically, it seems our brains – both individually and collectively – will not allow us to consider the possibility that our brain can show signs of illness.

Although my family has a strong medical background, I am not medically trained in any way. I took myself away from that path when I struggled to grasp the basic principles of science while studying as a teenager. However, I have asked myself, what surgical treatment can the medical profession provide for our brain?

In my humble opinion, there's not a huge amount that a top surgeon can do to the brain in the surgical theatre. In comparison, if someone has heart problems, there are numerous surgical procedures which can be carried out to fix the problem.

Whereas, due to the physical structure of our brain and its fragility, the option of patching things up surgically seems not to be realistic. Going back to the example of our heart, it is amazing to think that a surgeon and their team can stop our heart beating, mechanically carry out the function of our heart, fix the problem and start our heart beating again. That is truly amazing.

On the other hand, as far as I'm aware, once our brain stops working for any reason that is it: game over. The brain is in complete control of absolutely everything we do consciously. Our brain must operate well or we are worthless. I believe this is the conclusion which we have formed about the whole sphere of mental health, rightly or wrongly. None of us truly understand the magnificent splendor of our brain and everything it does.

This could be due to the common view that we only use 10% of our brain. Therefore, it is virtually impossible for us to even imagine what the other 90% does. Maybe it is this inherent lack of understanding and possible neglect which fuels the conclusion we have reached concerning mental health.

The conclusion that is reflected in the treatment provided for mental illness and our attitude towards it. We have thought treatment is satisfactory. Is it?

One of the greatest dilemmas surrounding mental health is that for someone to receive treatment, they must give their consent for the treatment to be carried out.

This is their right as a human being. However, when someone is suffering from mental ill health, the processes they go through in making any decision may be affected.

It may be glaringly obvious from someone on the outside looking in, that the decision to make is a simple one: to accept help, start on the road to recovery and stay on it until they are where they need to be, mentally.

However, if the person requiring treatment is not in the right frame of mind to make that decision, they can refuse to give their consent and not receive the treatment. This may often be the case when there is an official or unofficial dual diagnosis and the sufferer's demons are silently demanding their fix, but this is their right. Their suffering continues, as does the suffering of their family, loved ones and friends.

This is the tug of war that has been played out in the case of Stephen. The treatment is available and he may reluctantly accept it. He refuses to have the course of treatment, which the professionals believe will give him the long-term advantage over his illness. His attitude seems to be that as soon as the opportunity arises, he will walk away from the treatment. At that point, he will most likely feed the hunger he feels through his addictive personality and enter the revolving door, which will lead at some point straight back to hospital.

Here in the United Kingdom, the only way that you can be forced to accept treatment is if the police find you in such a poor state of mental health that you are posing a clear and present danger to yourself or to anyone else.

The treatment available is 'reactive' to the way someone comes across when faced by the police, or 'reactive' to their actions, which they have already carried out. Here's an example which illustrates the danger of this approach:

I live in a newly built house. My young family and I are the first residents to live here. As with any new build house there have been minor teething problems in addition to one potentially huge problem we experienced. There is an en-suite shower room, which my partner and I use. We also have a main bathroom, which the children use at bath time. They are normally supervised by my partner; otherwise by me. Both have huge mirrors, which run along almost the entire length of one of the walls. I guess they are around two to three metres square. The children have bath time most evenings prior to bedtime.

One evening, everything went as close to clockwork as possible in bathing and feeding before sleeping. It was the dead of night, I was just about ready to drift into a deep sleep, when I heard what I thought was the sound of an electrical fire. I ran out of the bedroom trying to locate the source of the sound. I paused in the hallway for a split second and thought

I must check my daughter's bedroom because I could see that my son was asleep in his bed through his open door.

As I took my first step towards my daughter's room, I heard what I perceived to be two explosions, followed by what sounded like debris hitting the bathroom door. I quickly checked my daughter and found her stirring, so I went back the couple of steps to the bathroom. When I opened the door, to my shock, I found that what I had imagined to be the electrical fire was the huge mirror peeling away from the wall. The explosions had been the mirror cracking under its own weight, before smashing onto the bath and floor where my children and partner had been only a few hours before. That mirror was so heavy I had to break it into three pieces the next morning to be able to move it and the glaziers – when they arrived within 48 hours of surveying the damage – carried the replacement as a team of three; made up of two people carrying the load with difficulty and one directing the load-bearers.

If we had known how weak the bond was between the wall and the mirror, there is no way that anyone would have been using either bathroom or shower room until they were strengthened. That is obvious. Waiting for what may be the inevitable to happen before seeking to fix the issue is 'reactive' and dangerous.

The police are not trained mental health workers. However, they are expected to make a potentially life or death decision when they are expected to judge whether someone they have encountered is of sound mind or not. That is how serious these situations can get, and how ridiculous the system's response is, maybe not only in this country, but throughout the world.

Also, it is not only a life and death decision for the person in front of the police, who may or may not be suffering. In very extreme cases, it could also be a life and death decision for the innocent bystander who could find themselves in the wrong place at the wrong time when the police have not noticed a condition, which they are not fully trained to recognise.

This means that the reactive nature of this approach is very dangerous for those suffering from the illness and for the public at large.

Although Stephen has never attacked anyone as a result of his illness, having witnessed his behaviour when his illness is at its height, it always reminds me of his agitated state when I arrived after he was attacked. I now believe he may have been experiencing one of his first episodes even then.

What about the treatment received by Stephen and all those people suffering while they are imprisoned voluntarily or involuntarily in the care system? It seems, looking from the outside in, that the care system aims to paper over the cracks. How do they achieve this aim? While in hospital, I have heard that the patients are filled with drugs relevant to the illness that the patient is perceived to have. As far as I am aware, that is it. Whether the patient is in hospital, voluntarily or through the legal process of being detained in hospital through the Mental Health Act, that seems to be all the help they receive – papering over the cracks. Once the patient is perceived to be fit enough to leave hospital, they are free to return to their semblance of a life and free to decide whether they want to continue with the medication, which barely helps them to continue - papering over the cracks.

They are free to decide whether they want to continue along the path of sustained recovery through therapy and other treatment potentially available, or to stray back onto the long or short path, which ultimately leads back to hospital or worse. In the case of dual diagnosis, when the addiction is not treated, it is sadly – as in Stephen's and likely most other cases – a matter of when, not if, they find themselves back in hospital.

That is the tightrope they walk even when they are not experiencing an episode or crisis. That is the cycle of life, which they live without proper, comprehensive, ongoing care treatment for all forms of mental ill health being provided by the system.

Stephen has been forcibly hospitalised on at least four occasions since 2010. Additionally, he has been admitted to hospital voluntarily on several occasions, and to be honest I have lost count of how many times we, or his home treatment staff, have had to report him missing.

Each time he has been out of hospital and on the right path for a long or short time, one thing or another has caused him to take the wrong path straight back to what seems to be square one.

I have come to learn that it is not only his illnesses, but also the hopeless inefficiency of the system, which allowed this to happen, fueled by misguided public attitude, lack of understanding, and lack of funding.

For the sake of the thousands and thousands of people going through the same mental torture, this really, really needs to change.

In desperately trying to get Stephen onto the right road to recovery and help Anna continue to make her recovery as strong as it can possibly be, my family and I have witnessed first-hand the extreme suffering which families go through when a loved one falls mentally ill. We can only try to imagine the mental and physical pain caused to the person suffering and the pain of the abuse they put themselves through.

Sometimes, the episodes of both loved ones have coincided, and has tested our resilience to the core. At other times, an episode for one has been almost instantly followed by an episode for the other. In trying to engage with the services available for them, I have witnessed the clear and heartbreaking reality that the so-called 'help' and care available for the sufferers is wholly inadequate.

That in a nutshell is my why.

- Why I am determined to help us all to change our innocent, but shameful, perception of mental illness.

- Why I am determined to make change for the better happen to the treatment available on a long-term basis, regardless of any obstacle.

- Why my family stand with me, one and all.

- And why I am determined that future generations, starting hopefully with our children, will view physical and mental health equally and should not have to go through the same degree of torture if they were to fall ill. If either of my children were to fall ill, I would never forgive myself if I knew that I had it within me to change the treatment available but had done nothing about it.

There is none of that excess baggage attached to mental health when someone has a physical ailment. I believe we need to view mental health in the same way so we can make the treatment available infinitely more effective through the plan I have devised through the Unity community.

In everything I do or experience, I always try to take any positive I can from every given situation or problem. Some people would view this as a strength, other people may view it as annoying to always draw positivity from any situation. I regard it as part of my nature. Life is made up of positives and negatives rather than strengths and weaknesses.

I have taken one of my positives and applied it to one of my negatives. This book is the result, and the plan it portrays is the positive result of that application. In a moment, I will ask you to consider what your three greatest positives and negatives are and make a note of them as a reminder to you of who you are. You may or may not take inspiration from the following example of the process.

One of your greatest positives may be that you are passionate. One of your negatives may be that you go through bouts of depression – an illness above anything else. If you were to decide to apply your passion to speaking out about depression with your family, among your friends, in your community, how much good could it do? You may help yourself by talking about it; you may help other people who suffer in silence to cope, by opening them up to the conversation; and you may inspire who knows how many other conversations, helping who knows how many other people. All of this by applying your positive to your perceived negative, which would ultimately make your negative shrink by having open two-way conversations during the lows.

In this section of our journey it should now be clear why I am taking on the task of challenging attitudes towards and improving treatment of mental health. Until this point, my personal journey has been inwards, discovering the conviction to take on this challenge due to my positives and negatives. For society to stand up to the mental health crisis in its midst, it also needs to look inwardly to find the root cause of the crisis.

Please take a moment now to consider; what are your greatest positives and negatives?

Chapter 4:
Where have I been and what have I learnt?

In this chapter, we will explore the inward journey I have been on since the loss of my father and the consequences of making hurried decisions with a clouded mind. We will then gain an insight into the positive and negative sides of my character, which have led to the profound importance of the message within this book, the plan it conveys and the change it will bring about.

In February 2008, I had to gain entry to my father's house only to find that I, and his fellow doctor colleague who was waiting outside, fearing the worst, had got there too late. As part of his profession, my father not only saved countless lives, but probably also brought as many, if not more lives into the world.

I may generalise here, but if you have ever tried to read a doctor's handwriting, it is a bit messy to say the least. My father's handwriting was exactly that, as were his organisational skills. But he was very highly thought of in his job as a consultant surgeon, although his life in general was complicated.

I had already given notice to leave work. My last day at work was due to be the day after the tragedy struck. My plan had been to travel for a short while and learn as I went. Learn how to live. However, I left work that day and instead of travelling I had to manage the affairs my father left. What I have come to learn about myself since his passing is so priceless to me that it must be shared.

Life, for a long time, was a bit like looking through a bubble. I realised that for the period of the immediate aftermath the enjoyable things in life would have to be put on hold while these several issues were dealt with. In the years after losing our father, my siblings and I had to make decisions that should not have been placed on us. I stand by some of those decisions – however unpopular they were – as I must. Other decisions, I believe were made with only heart breaking, painful emotion and impatience in mind; those which led to the worst consequences I went with against my gut feeling at the time. That will never happen again. I'm not saying they could never have been right, but with the sequence of events that followed, they were wrong decisions. If events hadn't happened as they did, we could have been right. Nothing any of us could have done in such incredibly complex circumstances would have changed the situation once the decisions were set. None of us involved in anyway were to blame for what unfolded.

Ultimately, that chain of events – of which there were many – following those decisions, indirectly and directly led to me having a successful petition for bankruptcy made against me in 2014. That bankruptcy was discharged one year later under law. I am now free from its financial grip. I have learnt that taking out credit and building up debt are not the way to living a happy life filled with fulfilment.

Thank you very much, but no thanks.

Filling the doughnut

The reason why I am thankful for being made bankrupt is not what you may think. Yes, supposedly my debts were written off and I was free to restart after one year with the bankruptcy being discharged. The reason for my gratitude towards those who dropped the axe and believed that I was doomed, is that they gave me a huge opportunity to fully survey the scene of my life and take priceless lessons from mistakes I had made to ensure they are never repeated. I initially had the seed planted for the ideas, which I now write about, around a year before my financial fate was sealed. Due to the incredibly complex circumstances surrounding my family, that seed has continued to grow since then, and is now ready to sprout its first leaf in the form of this book.

It has taken years of thinking for me to work out exactly what I have learnt. What triggered these thoughts? At one point, I ran my initial ideas past Ralph, a good friend of mine. He asked me a very important question.

'If I fell seriously ill, mate, how would you help me?'

I tried to respond to his question, but instantly realised there were too many holes in my answer. The answer to his question has been what I have been seeking and this book represents the filling in of the majority of those holes.

It took me considerable time to realise that life had to slow down to help me find them. Have you ever been so busy that you've not had time to stop, carrying on with the daily hustle and bustle of life in such a whirl that days turn into weeks seemingly in the blink of an eye? Then, as soon as you stop, you realise how quickly time has gone and that you've barely remembered to breathe.

*'The answers you seek never come when the mind is busy.
They come when the mind is still, when silence speaks loudest'*

Leon Brown – Baseball player, 1960s

I pondered Ralph's question for a period of time without making a huge amount of progress. I was trying to deal with too many other problems at once. Then I was lucky enough to get a job. My mind got busy again, concentrating on the job at hand while enjoying time with my partner and children when not working. But finding the answer to his question was always in the back of my mind.

In March 2014, I had to leave work again to help Stephen and Anna. Since then, when I've not been with my partner and children, I have been helping my extended family to cope with and recover from their illnesses. As the problems highlighted in Ralph's question have been all around me when I have been busy, when I do get chance to shut myself off from the outside world for a period of time, allowing my mind to be still, the answers start flooding in.

They have come from experiencing how I imagine countless families have to try to cope, witnessing what those suffering go through and being disgusted at how their treatment lets them down. This book gives you, the reader and the world at large, the answers.

The train of my thoughts

As you may or may not have already guessed, I have always been a bit of an introvert. Quite shy. I have always thought of this as a negative. However, I have learnt that it could be applied to a positive. What is an introvert? You may know a few? *The Huffington Post* states that: *'around a third to half of the population, are introverts... the truth is that many of our most prominent faces, past and present, have actually identified as introverts.'* (Ref. 2)

Please don't hold my admission against me. It turns out that I have something in common with some very well-known people. These include Bill Gates, Abraham Lincoln, Albert Einstein and J.K. Rowling.

Take J.K. Rowling, as an example. She first had the idea for the *Harry Potter* series while she was travelling alone on a long and delayed train journey from Manchester to London.

'I had been writing almost continuously since the age of six but I had never been so excited about an idea before.
To my immense frustration, I didn't have a pen that worked and I was too shy to ask anybody if I could borrow one.
I simply sat and thought, for four hours, while all the details bubbled up in my brain, and this scrawny, black haired, bespectacled boy who didn't know he was a wizard became more and more real to me.'

JK Rowling - author of the Harry Potter book series

Since I was young, I have had several good ideas, as most young lads do. While at University I had a perfect business idea, which I never acted on at the time. Some years later I took the idea to my father and we acted on it in the months before he passed away. Unfortunately, we were not in the right frame of mind to run this business in the aftermath of our loss, in addition to the huge decisions we had to endure, but we tried to carry on instead of taking more time to grieve. At the same time, we set up a separate business. This is one of the decisions, which I felt really uneasy about due to the timing. It could have worked. Against my gut feeling, we also tried to grow this second business far too quickly. During this period, we should have been grieving for my father, not taking on the world. This second business also failed. I think the saying goes; *'Once bitten, twice shy.'* I add to this: *'Three times and you're obsessively cautious!'*

When my quest for answers to Ralph's question really began to gather pace, I was facing the real possibility of my approaching bankruptcy. Like my father before me, I believe that laws are there for a reason. They have to be obeyed. Simple! I followed the bankruptcy restrictions to the letter. All financial activities were put on hold and I took every opportunity I possibly could to think and plan repeatedly, always with a sense of obsessive caution.

I feel the same sense of excitement about my seed, now. Additionally, like the bespectacled boy and the author's four-hour train journey, the seed which I planted some years ago, is now looking very healthy, having bubbled around in my brain for a long time. Through the support, which this book hopefully generates and your assistance, I hope this seed becomes a huge English oak tree. The time I have spent thinking and planning rather than doing over this time really has given it that potential to grow and thrive.

To understand the obsessive caution, which has governed my thought train, the best way to describe the process is to explain the checks and balances that are in place. We can do this by considering our instincts.

The head, heart and gut balancing act

During my long period of reflection, thought and planning, I tried to make sense of what my heart, my head and my gut were telling me.

The intuitive feelings that I got from each were often very different. An online article by Light Watkins, called *Seven surefire signs you're following your heart* (Ref. 5), helped me to relate his signs to the thought processes I had gone through to reaching where I am today. I want to share these with you, so you understand.

1. A heart message may not make sense to anyone, but you.

There are many directions in which my life could go right now. Those around me may think it would make perfect sense to carry on in the profession which I have been trained and excelled in, on and off for more than a decade. The only difference being, to work for myself on a flexi-time basis using my home as my base. While it is true that I am constrained to working for myself due to complex family responsibilities, I have no desire to pursue the path of working in that specific field any longer. Instead, by witnessing the suffering people go through and the day-to-day struggle their family endure in coping with the ailment and processing what is wrong with that, I feel compelled to follow the path I have chosen. This book is testament to that fact. My head has processed the information and my heart has taken control of what to do about the problems we have and that I have witnessed second hand.

2. There may be several unknown variables. You feel the call to try something big, but when you put your plan through a critical analysis, it has more holes than a doughnut shop. And yet, this doesn't seem to stop you.

My critical analysis started when I realised that I could not answer Ralph's question due to gaping holes. It did not stop me though. My heart told me to carry on and fill in the holes. With the assistance of several learned people, I think I have filled most of them at this point. Other holes may appear in the future, but I will continue regardless because my heart and the faith it holds, will command that I do so.

'Messages from our heart have no attached guarantees, and sometimes require enormous amounts of blind faith. As Martin Luther King, Jr. said, you don't need to see the entire staircase – just the first step.'

Light Watkins (Ref. 3)

Fortunately, the first step I have had to take is my head processing and following the commands from my heart. I have looked at all the gaping holes in my plan and processed the solutions which will fill them. Thought and planning over this long period of time, rather than doing, has given me that advantage. This has made it possible for me to show you what the first step is so you don't need as much blind faith to follow me through your heart's desire.

3. Heart-centred action can be scary, but in a good way.

I have always been inspired by the thought that if your dreams or aspirations do not scare you, they're not big enough. Every morning when I think about what I would like to achieve, I must admit that the thought of the adventure I wish to go on absolutely terrifies me but in a very, very good way. The great thing is that the only limits holding me back are those which I put in place.

In the short time that it takes us to complete this part of the journey, you should realise that my plan is virtually limitless in its potential. The only external limit will depend on the amount of public support I can generate. With that support in place, literally anything is possible.

4. Everyone (not just you) will benefit by your actions.

The whole of humanity is affected in some way or another by mental health.

'One in four people will be affected by mental or neurological disorders at some point in their lives. Around 450 million people currently suffer from such conditions, placing mental disorders among the leading causes of ill health and disability worldwide.
Treatments are available, but nearly two-thirds of people with a known mental disorder never seek help from a health professional
Where there is neglect, there is little or no understanding.
Where there is no understanding, there is neglect.'

The World Health Organisation, 2001 (Ref. 4)

The 450 million are assumed to be people who have seen specialists, been diagnosed and accept the fact they are ill to some degree, suffering from an invisible affliction. How many other people are there in the world who may be ill and they don't realise it? Even more frightening is that the 450 million people may only represent a third of the real number. If you factor in their families who are also affected and their friends who also witness the suffering, that is near enough everyone on the planet.

These figures are from the turn of the millennium. Are we just more aware of mental ill health now or is this increased awareness mirrored by occurrence globally of mental ill health? If so, it is horrifying to imagine what the true figure is today, more than 15 years on. Therefore, the whole of humanity will benefit from the changes I seek to bring about. On a personal level, my duty is to instill all of our human basic core values in my children and ensure they have the best, most comfortable start to their life journey as possible. That is my only personal motivation, not personal gain.

As Light Watkins suggests, true heart messages *are rooted in the process of generosity, compassion, love, cooperation, communication, forgiveness and empathy.'* These are the driving forces pushing this plan forward, in combination with my heart's burning desire to make it happen.

5. Immediate action is required. Heart messages require real-time responses. They are not concerned with the past, the future or even with details about the present. Whether you feel you have enough money, resources, or influence is irrelevant to your heart. If you let those perceived shortcomings stop you from following through, you may miss your window of opportunity.

My greatest fear has been that the window of opportunity Watkins refers to will slam shut. I have learnt that I am holding the window open with my determination to make things happen.

There have been many distractions, but the focus required by my heart's demands remains strong. For example, I have had almost no money, apart from what is needed for the bare essentials required to exist. I have worked with limited resources such as, believe it or not, a very unreliable internet connection. And my influence has been limited by the need to provide for my family and children, but my heart is still in control.

6. A heart message is about what's right, not what's wrong.

Watkins believes that it is your heart which gives you the right direction to take in life. Sometimes there may be alarm bells, which make you shy away from taking a particular path. This, he believes, is your gut telling you that a particular decision may or would be wrong. Paying attention to both is very important, as I have learnt from not listening to my gut in the past, but I will never do that again.

7. It feels like the right thing to do.

There is an important reason why I am telling you so much about myself and the processes I have been through. If I were to come straight out with what I want to do, without explaining what has driven me to take this path, how and why I believe it is so necessary, you would probably think I am in need of having my own head examined. Throughout this long period of planning with obsessive caution, I have discovered the majority of the answers I needed to answer Ralph's question with confidence.

'Employ your time in improving yourself by other men's writings so that you shall gain easily what others have labored hard for.'

Socrates – Greek Philosopher

This book and the project it represents are the result of going back to the drawing board hundreds of times. This is only the start. The benefits for humanity could be limitless. When enough people take even the smallest bit of something resembling inspiration from what I write, then the vision I will show you will become my life's success.

Watkins concludes that our hearts tell us what is right, while our guts tell us what is wrong. In addition to this, I believe our heads act as the fail-safe, processing messages prior to action. I also believe our head can override our heart and our gut. If our head is not in the right place when making decisions that can affect our life in immeasurable ways, then our heart and our gut can be rendered obsolete. This can truly lead to meltdown, both physically and mentally.

When you have read this book, I hope beyond hope that your heart comes out on top and your head tells you to go with it; there's nothing to lose and everything to gain for humanity's sake! Everything that you read in this book comes from my heart. The determination to make change happen is also deeply rooted in my soul.

Make yourself a promise today – no matter how big or small – write it down and let your inner circle of family and friends know about your promise. Back that promise with undying determination to make it happen come what may and the world could be your oyster. Believe!

PART TWO:
WE

Chapter 5:
Who are we?

Have you ever been on your way to do something, whether it is at home or at work, got to where you should be to carry out that task and completely forgotten what it was you were going to do? To put your mind at rest, I'm not talking about a major task here, just one of those mundane things you probably do on a daily basis. We are going to explore the solution to this problem and apply it to modern day life.

My partner, our two children and I have dinner together every evening, almost without exception. My partner is a great cook and she does the majority of the cooking. I am in charge of getting the table set with cutlery, condiments and the children sat up to the table, ready to eat. This is quite a task. We have an open plan kitchen and lounge, so this all takes place in the one room. My partner orchestrates proceedings and reminds me of anything I've forgotten to do. The requests from the children come in thick and fast. I can sometimes find my head spinning. I find myself in the kitchen or at the table, thinking what on earth did I come here to get or to do? I pause for a second and do not have the answer to hand. So, what do I do?

If you find yourself in this same position at any time, then I recommend you give this a try.

I go back to exactly where I have just come from. This may be to one of my children who I was attending to last, or back to the dining table.

Normally within a split second I have realised exactly what I was supposed to do or get, and I go back and do it or get it without a second hesitation. Re-visiting where I have come from always yields the answer. This also worked in the lightning quick office atmosphere I used to work in.

Do we know who we are and why we are here?

When we, the human race, popped up on this planet, tens of thousands or so years ago, we came in way down the pecking order and lived in the shadows of the creatures that ruled the earth. We were and still are animals; mammals, to be exact. We formed part of the food chain and it was a matter of survival when we were the prey of the earth's rulers. Our primary functions were to eat, sleep, drink water, breathe and reproduce. Those were the only functions we had to fulfill to survive. When you consider, we were probably somewhere in the mid to lower end of the food chain, we must have carried out those functions pretty well because we are still here today.

Through luck, intelligence, learning, natural law in being Darwin's 'fittest', and mainly acting as one unified group, we have forced our way very, very quickly up to now being the kings and queens of the earth. Now we, the human race, rule the world and everything in it. We are now – rightly or wrongly – at the top of the food chain looking down on every other creature inhabiting the earth. On the face of it, we must still be eating, sleeping, drinking water, breathing and reproducing very well. The best we could possibly be. Surely, that must be the case?

To be frank, yes, we are still doing very well. We eat as well as we have ever done. Surely, there is nothing edible on earth that we haven't tried and made into a delicious, nutritious meal. We drink so much water that we now bottle it. Everyone currently on earth is still living, breathing and sleeping, otherwise they wouldn't be here and we are reproducing at an astonishing rate. The human population inhabiting the earth is now more than seven billion people.

Are you satisfied with my answer to the last question I raised?

Am I? No!

But why?

Why do I feel uneasy at leaving that answer where it is? Care to join me in seeing why?

If you are prone to triggers of anxiety, panic or depression, it may be best to skip to Part Three at this point.

The choice is yours.

What follows may be a sharp dose of reality.

Only read what follows in this section with great care because it could make your adventure; that of your children; or even your grandchildren all the more enjoyable, if you are...

- A youngster looking forward to leaving school and setting out on this great adventure called life.

- A couple thinking of trying for your first child and considering the great adventure that will bring.

- A couple who have children and are already enjoying the adventure of parenthood.

- A couple with grownup children and reveling in the adventure of being a grandparent.

'The Earth is 4.6 billion years old.
scaling that to 46 years, humans have been here for four hours,
the industrial revolution began one minute ago
and in that time, we have destroyed more
than half the world's forests.'

Greenpeace

Without being fully-fledged environmentalists, the above quote is a little bit scary. Don't you agree? If we continue along the same path for another minute, does that mean there would be no forests left on earth?

Going further into the environmental issues this raises, the problems we are seeking to provide an answer to on our journey are not environmental. We need to understand that the environment, which surrounds us – as with the environmental factors which play a role in Stephen's illness – could be, in every sense, a big part of the mental health crisis we face. Let's consider our basic human needs: breathing, drinking water, eating, sleeping and reproducing.

How well are we breathing?

We all live on earth. If the earth were a human body and the trees, which formed the forests we have destroyed and those that remain would be similar to our lungs. If the earth had two lungs like us, we have taken one of them away.

The trees help the Earth – our collective home – to breathe. If we get ill, our temperature goes up and we get what's called a fever. So the Earth has a fever, it's getting hotter. When we get ill, our body fights off what makes us ill using our immune system. The Earth's immune system is a layer of gas, which surrounds the Earth miles up in the sky above us. By allowing the Earth to breathe, the trees play a major role in keeping the Earth's immune system working – getting rid of the bad and keeping the good in the air which we breathe. While all of this is happening in the sky above us, what are we doing?

There are seven billion humans on Earth. Almost absolutely everything we do down here, causes gases to be blown out into the air and into the sky, high, high above us and above the blue sky and clouds, which we can see. For example, if there are seven billion of us down here, how many cars are there? There must be billions. Each and every car is giving the air we breathe a good dose of not very nice gas.

As the Earth is feeling a little bit rough and has a fever while it's immune system isn't working very well, we're stuck down here breathing it all in. From the car exhausts, the airplane engines, the chimneys and so on. So how's our breathing at the moment? Not great? We must consider the strong point that the wellbeing of our mind and body is harmonious in its interconnection. What if the air that we breathe is not only affecting our lungs, therefore our body, but also, possibly our mental health too. Experts have begun to show their grave concern in this area:

'A major new study has linked air pollution to increased mental illness in children, even at low levels of pollution'

The Guardian newspaper online (Ref. 5)

So, why do we allow it to continue?

How good is what we drink?

The fact that we have polluted the environment and the air we breathe so much that the Earth has a fever and is heating up, means the huge areas of ice at the northern and southern most tips of the Earth are melting. This melting produces water, which flows into the seas making sea levels rise and areas of land very close to sea level are under real threat of flooding. According to the USGS, the US science agency for a changing world, established by an act of congress in 1879 within the Department of the Interior, *'About 71% of the Earth's surface is water covered.'* (Ref. 6)

The threat is real and it's staring us in the face if we live on low-lying land close to the sea and on islands. If we were to view a continent as being a very big island, that means this problem is staring each and every one of us directly in the face. And yet, way back when we humans first popped up, one of our basic human functions helping us to survive was drinking water.

A chemistry expert, Anne Marie Helmenstine, Ph.D, in March 2017, stated that the amount of water that makes up the human body ranges from 50-75% (Ref. 7). On average, an adult body is 50-65% water, whereas, an infant's body is 75-78% water. Yet despite the fact that we, and the Earth, are predominantly made up of water, there is serious lack of water available.

'783 million people do not have access to clean water and almost 2.5 billion do not have access to adequate sanitation.
6 to 8 million people die annually from the consequences of disasters and water-related diseases.'

United Nations, World Water Day 2013 (Ref. 8)

As a result, there are way too many people who die every year in areas that were arguably first exploited and then left neglected. These human beings are dying from a serious lack of drinking water. The water that is available for these human beings to drink is so disease ridden that it is deadly poisonous, but they and their children have to drink it. There have been reports that even in America there are serious concerns about the lack of water on the West Coast.

We may over-simplify the point, but hopefully we will not miss the point. Surely, a huge clue to the solution to this problem is that the coastal areas are suffering from drought. If anyone living in that location looked west from high ground, they would see billions of tonnes of water in the sea.

'The oceans hold about 96.5% of all Earth's water.'

USGS (Ref. 6)

I know the sea is made up of salt water. And? The 'and?' is a bit of a problem here, because the 'and' is all the pollutants and rubbish which have got into the sea due to our hard work and the natural biological waste caused by the creatures which inhabit the sea.

There have been numerous solutions to this problem suggested. One was provided by a Dutch teenager Boyan Slat, aged 19, who designed a machine to clean the sea removing man made materials from the sea (Ref. 9). What if the invention could be further modified to remove the harmful toxins by pumping salt water through a cleaning filter before boiling off the salt and storing what's left as pure drinking water? These and other ideas are brilliant and could save millions of lives by discovering an almost limitless supply of drinking water, which is getting bigger by the day due to the melting ice.

Bravo! Truly genius!

The inventor may have saved millions of human beings from dying of dehydration through lack of drinking water or having to drink poisonous water or flooding. The solutions to the biggest problems we human beings experience, are quite often staring us in the face, along with the problems in question. Sustainable supplies of drinking water have become a big problem for a big part of the human race, but this is one of our basic human functions, which we need to survive. But what else do we drink as well as water to quench our thirst? The answer is sugar.

The drinks we consume on a daily basis are laden with sugar. Even when we buy fruit juice, it has an unhealthy amount of sugar in it. The measurable affects this has on the body, in the form of diabetes, heart disease, obesity and other health complications, is enormous. For years now, there has been growing concern about an impending obesity epidemic throughout the western world. This has now grown to such a degree that the American Heart Association in August 2015, stated that one in three US adults is obese (Ref. 10).

> *'...predictions that half of the British population will be obese by 2050 'underestimate' the scale of the obesity crisis.'*

UK Telegraph newspaper online (Ref. 11)

In the documentary film called *Fed Up. It's Time to Get Real About Food* Stephanie Soechtig, presents overwhelmingly strong evidence that the major driving force behind obesity is sugar consumption (Ref. 12). The as-yet unmeasured knock-on effect this consumption could have on our mind is as big if not bigger. Have you ever experienced the seemingly euphoric sensation of a 'sugar rush'? Many of our children experience this almost every day. It is argued that the low following the high of a sugar rush can cause anxiety and depression or at the very least copy the symptoms. Not good!

> *'Science has proven that sugar is one of the*
> *most chemically addictive substances, but there*
> *are also psychological issues with sugar consumption,*
> *especially for those who have addictive tendencies.*
> *It is a comfort, it is a rush, it is a sense of escape.*
> *It's not hard to see why so many people are addicted to sugar.'*

Tim Stoddart – co-founder and current president of Sober Nation (Ref. 13)

A big question arises that we must ponder at this point. Specialists argue that consumption of sugar has the same effect on the brain as what we call class A drugs. By allowing children to feast on so much sugar, are we allowing them to take their first step towards addiction and mental health problems? There have been several films produced focusing on the hidden dangers of sugar, and added sugar in foods we assume do not contain sugar.

A report produced by Public Health England – the agency in charge of the nation's health - has recommended a possible tax on the sale of products high in sugar content. The money raised from this tax would be put towards the huge cost of treating the illnesses which obesity causes. The report and its suggestions and recommendations were initially dismissed by the government.

The era of artificial sweeteners started decades ago. We humans, at heart, have a 'sweet tooth'. We cannot get enough of the sweet stuff. Artificial sweeteners provided the means to have as much sweet as we want without any of the bad effects on our health. Brilliant, we thought, let's feast on the artificially sweet drinks and stay healthy at the same time. This couldn't be better!

There have been numerous arguments linking these artificial sweeteners to varying serious illnesses, including links to mental ill health in the form of depression and its associates. However, it seems that once again we have buried our head in the sand and ignored the warning signs or dismissed them as wrong.

How on earth can anything so good, be bad for you? Being our collective conclusion. 'It doesn't hurt me when I drink it so what's the worry' has been our collective response. 'The kids can drink it by the bucket load too as they'll get the sweet taste but it will do them no harm.'

Really?

What if the arguments are even partly right?

The same and even more can be said about alcohol which is proven to kill in high enough doses, if sustained for long enough, although it doesn't directly affect our children. Does it? Why continue to drink anything artificially sweetened, arguably or even proven to be dangerous, when it could be affecting our body and mind?

A great deal of what we drink or could drink is very healthy, especially when it is produced as close as possible to its natural state, such as fresh juices that we juice ourselves. To be guaranteed to be natural, probably best to have grown it in the garden too.

The lack of pure drinking water is either killing millions of us through lack of availability, or harming our collective body and mind through the possible addition of chemicals. At the same time, what we do have available to drink is doing as much if not more harm through its sugar, artificial and alcoholic content.

How well do we eat?

Now, on to the main course. As the saying goes: *'You are what you eat.'*

'When scientists study feelings, they start out by looking for something to measure. They draw up scales for suicidal tendencies, test hormone levels to measure love or trial tablets to treat anxiety. To outsiders, this often appears less than romantic.

In Frankfurt, there was even a study which involved scanning the brains of volunteers while a research assistant tickled their genitals with a toothbrush.

Such experiments tell scientists which areas of the brain receive signals from which parts of the body. This helps them draw a map of the brain…

Signals from the gut can reach different parts of the brain, but they can't reach everywhere. For example, they never end up in the visual cortex at the back of the brain.

If they did, we would see visual effects or images of what is going on in our gut. Regions they can end up in, however, include the insula, the limbic system, the prefrontal cortex, the amygdala, the hippocampus and the anterior cingulate cortex.

Any neuroscientists will be up in arms when I roughly define the responsibilities of these brain regions as respectively, self-awareness, emotion, morality, fear, memory, and motivation. This does not mean that our guts control our moral thinking, but it allows for the possibility that the gut might have a certain influence on it.'

Giulia Enders – author, *Gut: The Inside Story of Our Body's Most Underrated Organ, Scribe UK, 2015* (Ref. 14)

As Enders suggests, it could be that the way we look after our gut may have an effect on our mental wellbeing. This is highlighted when Enders features in her book a study, which concluded that the test animals who were fed bacteria known to be good for their gut function, heavily out performed those with normal or depressive tendencies. One of the biggest networks of nerves present in the human body runs messages between the gut and the brain. When the same network was disabled in the test animals highlighted, all the animal participants reverted to normal performance.

The food we eat directly affects the levels of 'good and bad' bacteria in our guts (Ref. 15). Anna has suggested to me on many occasions that she eats according to her emotions. What if the food we eat could be affecting our mental health?

Way back when we humans popped up on Earth, and since then, we have been and are omnivores. We will eat other kinds of animals and plants: meat, vegetables, leaves and grains of various kinds. During those times, the food we ate was either natural plants or wild animals. And we were natural and wild.

The type of food that we now eat has never been so plentiful and varied. However, alarm bells start to get louder and louder the closer the food gets on its journey from the farm or factory and through the way it is produced these days, all ready to heat and eat. Yummy!

During my mid-teenage years, I remember there was a food scare, which almost put me off eating a particular type of meat forever. The scare turned out to be the result of the way the animals which produced the meat had been fed. They were given feed which made them seriously ill and that tainted meat got into our human food supply. It lead to the debilitating disease being passed on to a number of people who, in turn suffered from a similar crippling, terminal disease called C.J.D. The disease which the animals got was known as Mad Cow Disease. From memory, that feeding method was only used in the United Kingdom and so the health problems were not global, but it goes to show what a devastating affect tampering with the food chain can have.

That method of feeding obviously ceased as soon as we became aware of the illness and its causes. However, it may have been said at the time that the number of sufferers may not be truly known for years to come because the onset of the disease could be years after consuming the meat.

What happens to the food we eat today before it reaches our table? Now, we are not food scientists, we may possibly exaggerate a little bit here, but don't worry too much, let's hope it is an exaggeration and if it is then it's only for effect.

If you were asked if you'd like to eat dangerous chemicals, would you be tempted? Let's consider the vegetables, leaves and grains which we eat and remember the food chain. We grow these crops for our own consumption. There are other creatures, which form part of the food chain, who also eat these types of food. I'm thinking mainly of insects. We call them pests. So we have devised a way of fixing the pest problem. We spray the vegetables, leaves and grains with chemicals, which either make the food taste so disgusting to the pests that they don't eat them or – and this is the more likely outcome – the pests are killed when they come into contact with or eat these chemicals.

Our food is safe to continue on its journey towards our dining table without being stolen by the pests.

Now, for another question!

Would we be willing to take part in an experiment to see whether these chemicals are harmful to us?

No, thanks!

We should understand at this point that there would be other ways to test if these chemicals are harmful to our long-term health, but such tests could not be done over the course of a lifetime. Even if they could be tested over a lifetime, we wouldn't be eating it while waiting for the test results and by the time the results came out it would be too late. As a result, there's no way of knowing the true cost we pay in terms of the effect on our body and mind, by eating vegetables, leaves and grains that are grown in this fashion. There are numerous arguments that these chemicals are affecting our body and our mind. Oh well, we could give up the greens and only eat meat instead!

Let's check out the meat on special offer. But before we do, how are the animals fed today before reaching our table? There is a strong possibility that the animals are fed on very similar if not the same grains, which we eat in one form or another. So we can assume the grain and other feed they are given has been treated with the chemicals we are exposed to in eating our greens.

If it is even partly correct that the greens we eat are affecting us, then the same may be true for the meat we eat. What if the meat is being tainted in the same way that caused Mad Cow Disease and we don't know it yet? What effect could this be having on our overall physical and mental health?

In addition, much of the meat which we and our children eat is processed. A Google search defines processed meat as below.

'Processed meat is defined as a meat product containing no less than 300g/kg meat, where meat either singly or in combination with other ingredients or additives, has undergone a method of processing other than boning, slicing, dicing, mincing or freezing, and includes manufactured meat.'

There are three words or phrases in that definition, which stand out and scream, alarm bells!

Firstly, *'300g/kg'* - that means three hundred grams per kilogram. Right, now let's rewind slightly.

'...processed meat is defined as a meat product containing no less than 300g/kg meat...'

If we're eating a burger, sausage or whatever, we assume we are eating something which is in large part, meat. We are wrong, by the unofficial definition above. It can be as little as a third meat. So what on earth is the rest made up of?

Secondly, *'additives'* which it seems make up more than two thirds of the sausage, burger or whatever processed rubbish it is. You can imagine. But a good part of the additives is most likely to be more chemicals and flavour enhancers such as our very good friend sugar.

We all know that salt is not good for you. Do you remember why? Well it's not good for you because the chemical salt, or sodium chloride causes high blood pressure, which is bad. But high blood pressure can lead to heart disease, which is even worse. Both are killers. Salt is classed as a food additive.

Another food additive, which may or may not be added to processed meat, but is used almost as much as salt, is MSG or Monosodium Glutamate. There have been studies, which indicate that this chemical – used as a flavour enhancer – is also bad for us physically and mentally.

For example, we must remind ourselves of the dream described at the very beginning of this book? While growing up and to this day, I will occasionally have a take away meal. There is one specific type of take away available worldwide – not a specific meal but a whole menu – in which almost every dish you could order is (not literally) full of MSG.

Ever since I was a young lad, if I ever have that type of take away for dinner, I always have the weirdest, most life-like dreams that night. Isn't it odd that what we eat can affect our mind and even our subconscious in that manner? For example, I'm pretty sure I had one such take away on the night I had the dream about my father.

Thirdly, the problem we should all have with *'manufactured meat'* as the definition states is do we really know what we're eating? Let's consider a shocking example.

A couple of years ago there was another food scandal in the UK, which rocked parts of the European Union when it came to light in the news. You probably heard about it. There were some well-known food manufacturers who were providing pre-packed, ready-made frozen meals such as spaghetti bolognese and lasagne. Somehow, when these meals were routinely tested and checked in a laboratory by scientists, they were found to contain not only beef but traces of horse meat! You wouldn't believe it would you? Horse meat in meals that kids love to eat. It is likely the majority of our children love to eat such as lasagne etc. especially when processed so it can be warmed in minutes by a microwave. Given the choice, my children prefer these types of meal homemade with love, when their mother has time to do so.

How do we know what effect the food we eat is having on our body and mind when we don't even know for sure, exactly what we are eating?

The same can be said for the whole idea of 'manufactured meat.' From memory, it may have once been jokingly called *'Anything goes'* meat or better, 'anything goes into it meat.' Literally anything! So long as that *'Anything'* is all from the same animal that's ok. Is it?

Really?

The same principle was used in feeding cows in the UK leading to the Mad Cow Disease. Look what happened to the cows and those poor human beings who became infected.

Add to the above the amount of sugar and fatty foods we eat and we give to our children. What effect is it having on them?

There are currently more obese people in the world than there have ever been. That disease is harming not only their body, but also their mind, when they become depressed about their body size and yet it continues.

Why?

> *"You know, I know this steak doesn't exist.*
> *I know that when I put it in my mouth,*
> *'The Matrix' is telling my brain that it is juicy and delicious.*
> *After nine years, you know what I realise? ...Ignorance is bliss."*

The Matrix (Ref. 16)

Food is measurably having a huge effect on our collective body. It could also be having an immeasurable effect of equal or greater proportion on the collective mind. Not only of our current generation but also of the next generation and however many generations follow after that.

But it tastes great and it doesn't affect us in the present tense, so let's carry on eating it.

Why?

If the saying is true in another sense that; *'We are what we eat'*, then like the processed meat and the mix of chemicals we consume, we are truly mixed up and, as in the case of Mad Cow Disease, messed up emotionally and physically, in mind and body.

Why do we carry on along the same path?

How are we sleeping?

When we eat well, we become tired. This is due to the energy we use in digesting our food. How do we sleep once we drift off?

Life as we know it has become like a merry-go-round speeding at a thousand miles per hour. When Stephen suffers from a manic episode caused by his illness, he can go for literally days on end without sleep. His mental state gets increasingly worse as his time without sleep increases.

Generally, the way we sleep reflects the stresses and strains of daily life. For example: Get up; get dressed; eat; shout at the children and have fun with them in unequal measure; kids to school; go to work; treat other people or be treated unkindly whilst wearing a smile; travel home packed in like a sardine; try to expel work issues from your mind; pick up the children; shout at the children and have fun in unequal measure; cook dinner; have dinner either together or in separate rooms or together but staring at the television; play time with the children or homework depending on their age; children ready for bed; play time and shouting in equal measure; children to bed; up; bed; up; bed; children asleep; stare at television; go to bed; bills in mind; try to sleep; deadline at work; try to sleep; debts; try to sleep, this problem, try to sleep, that problem, try to sleep, the other problem, try to sleep; don't try to sleep; fall asleep; alarm, wake up; and repeat all the above. Another day and another.

In today's dog-eat-dog world, sleep has become a priceless commodity. Sleeping for around six to eight hours a night allows our mind and body to recharge so we are ready to take on the challenges of the day ahead of us with energy levels and vitality at full strength. Being able to relax and sleep has become so difficult for a big portion of humanity, that chemicals are used to induce what may seem to be a good night's sleep. But due to those chemicals still being in our blood stream the next day, we are not full of energy; and vitality is hard to come by. So we turn to energy drinks – more sugar, more chemicals and more caffeine – not good for our mind or our body, but it helps to get us through the day. We need to take a break.

The reproductive spiral

Are we passing on the effects of what we take in at the point of conception? What if we are passing the effects of what we breathe, eat and drink on to the next generation before they are born?

Remember that Stephen's condition has genetic factors, which it is possible he could have been born with. Evolution is an advantage but also a disadvantage here. Animals evolve in such a way as to make survival as easy as possible. In this sense, as we, the human race evolve, maybe we are doing so in such a way as to protect us from the damage we are doing to ourselves. This might be the up side. On the down side, we could be evolving in such a way that makes us more vulnerable to sensitivity, not only in our body, but also in our mind, mainly as a result of the as-yet unknown effects of the chemicals we are exposed to on a daily basis.

Everything that we do daily, which we consider to be our basic human functions just could be leaving us wide open to disease in our collective body and illness of the mind, absolutely everything we do. It could be that deep down, we are aware of this. Living the *'ignorance is bliss'* approach; ignoring all the signs to be wary of the path we are on.

'The body cannot live without the mind.'

The Matrix (Ref. 16)

It is our collective mind that we must be concerned about in two senses. First, there are millions of people whose mind is literally torturing them through mental illness. Second, the rest of us are ignoring their plight. We are also ignoring the possibility that it is the way we live and the basic human functions which we carry out to survive that are making us, the human race, ill in the mind.

We need to work out why we seem to be living with our heads buried in the sand.

Ponder for a moment, who are the most important people in your life and the objects which you place most value on?

Chapter 6:
The "I Collective"

In the last section, we were left with a number of questions to answer relating to our basic human functions. To refresh our memory, these questions were as follows.

- Why do we continue to pollute our home, Earth, to such an extent that the air we and our children breathe may be affecting our mind and body while causing our home, Earth, to show worrying signs of decline?

- Why do we continue to produce food in such a way that it may well be having a very negative effect on our mind and body?

- Why do we allow millions of people to die each year through lack of clean drinking water, while at the same time, we and our children drink sugar like there's no tomorrow and do so watching the sea levels rise at an alarming rate?

- Why do we continue to live life at such a stressful pace that it's stopping us from sleeping properly, affecting us mentally and physically?

- Why are we not terrified about the fact that we could be passing on the way we have polluted ourselves and our planet, to our children before they are even born?

In this chapter, we will discover the probable answer to all these questions, remembering that we need to do so from our hearts.

Without wishing to be overly critical or harsh, it is actually the way that we as a human race are living, collectively, which is the huge issue here. In the last 'minute' since the Industrial revolution, we have logically progressed to where we are now, but we have to realise that there are serious physical and mental consequences for the way we are living. This is what needs attention.

Are you ready for the answer to the questions posed above?

There is a simple, one word answer, but the issues it raises run very deep and could ultimately destroy the world we live in, after it has firstly destroyed our minds completely.

That word is money.

Everything we do in the current world revolves around money. Even our basic human functions now involve money. The example we should consider here is water. Drinking water, which we have to do to survive, involves money. We must not moan about this fact of life, but we have to pay to have water, to drink water, to use water, whether it's from the tap or a bottle.

If we were to travel way back in time to meet some original people and somehow get across to them the concept of money and that we have to pay to drink water, I'm sure they would give us a look as if to say we're crazy. If we carried on and told them how everything else works; we'd probably be sent to their version of what we now call a mental institution!

Anyway, back to the important points we need to consider. Money is now our life. Here are several examples, which I am sure we all have heard many times:

- I've got no money!

- I need money to survive!

- I'm not happy!

- I've got loads of money!

- I want more money!

- I will not be happy until I've got loads more money!

- Then, I'll still want more money and I will not be happy until I get more money.

- I want this. I want that.

- I want everything that I've not got. Once I've got everything I will still want more.

- I will use something until it's useless, then in an instant I'll get rid of it.

- I want an upgrade. Where's my upgrade? I want it now!

- I don't want to queue up why should I have to queue up!

- When I've finished with anything, I will throw it away. Someone else can be paid to pick it up. That's how considerate I am.

- How much do I owe? Too much I know!

- But I must keep going, keep going, keep going, I must!

- I am a perfectionist; everything has to be absolutely perfect. I can't understand why I'm never happy with life.

- I eat processed food because it's all I can afford.

- I eat at the best restaurants and get the best food that money can buy! I want more!

- I will eat until I'm full but I will eat more anyway because I can.

Stop!

At this point, let's see what our old friend Socrates had to say about food.

> *'Worthless people live only to eat and drink;*
> *People of worth eat and drink only to live.'*

Socrates – Greek Philosopher

We are ironically *'eating and drinking'* ourselves towards our own destruction. Everything in the current world is about *'how much I can get'* or *'how can I get more.'*

This applies to anything and everything, whether it's a house, a car, clothes, everything. The means to get absolutely everything we want materially in life, but what we are never ultimately happy with, is money. Once we've got it, it is consumed in one way or another and we're still not happy so we go out and get more to consume. This is the age of consumption and it is through this consumption we are self-destructing.

Could it be possible that in our subconscious, our dreams or somewhere in the 90% of the brain we may not understand, we are aware that what we are doing will lead to our own destruction, and that is what is making the world so anxious, depressed and panic ridden?

Whatever it is, we continue on regardless, on our path towards self-destruction. This is similar to how someone who suffers from mental illness cannot seem to stop their actions in causing their own self-destruction; it is part and parcel of the illness as witnessed through the pain and suffering of Stephen and Anna.

All-consuming addiction

Addiction and mental illness go hand in hand. Whether it is in someone's nature to become ill, or whether they are nurtured towards it by their environment, is a question for professional psychologists. In this case, we should question whether nature and nurture also go hand in hand leading us towards the same fate. For example, the addictive nature of the sugar-laden food and drink, which we consume in vast quantities has lead us unwittingly down the path towards addiction. Arguably this takes place from a very young age when you consider the amount of sugar our children consume. We could put it down to what's called an addictive personality.

'Addiction depends, first and foremost, upon having an addictive personality. Such people, estimated at perhaps 10–15% of the population, simply don't know when to stop.'

Stephen Mason PhD – psychologist, former university professor, syndicated newspaper columnist and radio talk-show host

What if this underestimates the percentage of the population with an addictive personality? Is it reasonable to argue that any form of obsessive behavior could be even partly related to having an addictive personality?

'An addictive personality is a set of personality traits that make an individual more prone to develop addictions to drugs, alcohol or other habit forming behaviors.'

Natalie Baker – USA Psychotherapist

Let's consider the point raised by Natalie Baker, that an addictive personality can also relate to any of our habits, widening the goal posts considerably. There are common elements among people with varying addictions that relates to personality traits. People who are substance dependent are characterised by a physical or psychological dependency that negatively affects their quality of life.

However, people with addictive personalities are also highly at risk of becoming addicted to gambling, food, pornography, exercise, work and codependency.

Is what we consume from a very young age leading us all to develop an addictive personality from childhood? Could it be? We have a serious problem here and the sooner we realise that and collectively seek to solve this problem, the sooner we can get back to enjoying life and live it the way we would like to; in the more natural way we are supposed to.

But what is the problem?

Going back to my original point in answering the questions raised in the last section, absolutely everything we do revolves around money. Do you remember the outline of a typical day when referring to how we don't sleep so well anymore? That was an extreme form of how we might imagine a typical family day. Hectic.

The adults go to work to get as much money as possible, so the family can collectively consume as much as possible. The children are at school learning skills, which the parents hope will give them the means to earn as much money as possible, so they can consume more than the parents have been able to provide, once they too are grown up. We must consider whether that is living life to the full, or just existing.

Where is the quality of life in that mode of living? There is no quality of life, but it doesn't matter as it is all about the money! All we seem to live for in the present tense is money. That is what takes parents away from their children for the whole day and steals those precious moments from both parents and children. The pursuit of more money, which can be spent on consuming as much as we possibly can, simply to want more and more and more, and never being happy with exactly what is in front of us when we wake up each morning; our partner and children.

But we have to go out and get more. Just like an addict needs their fix. Our blinkered, non-stop pursuit of money is leading us down the path towards our own self-destruction. We are showing all the signs of being addicted to money and everything we can get with it. If we have no money we will do whatever we have to, with the aim of getting some money. If we have money, we want more and more, no matter the consequences in terms of our health or the health of the planet, our home.

All we need to do to break the momentum is realise that life does not, should not, and cannot revolve only around money. But we cannot and will not until we break out of the 'I Collective' that shackles us to money as its slave.

However, I believe that we can break these shackles, by asking ourselves a simple question and answering it honestly.

Ready?

Is what we're doing and the way we're living sane or insane?

In answering that question honestly, let's take into consideration what we've just discovered.

Mental illness can make the mind become self-destructive, leading to the sufferer taking self-destructive actions in many guises. Addiction in its most lethal form will ultimately lead to the self-destruction of the sufferer because they do not stop in their pursuit of whatever it is they feel they need, no matter who they hurt or what they destroy, even if it is themselves. This is their plight.

> *'Insanity is... doing the same thing over and over again and expecting different results.'*

Albert Einstein – Physicist

These are very wise words to ponder at this point. Let's consider this as we look at the way we are living with the knowledge we now have. Mental health problems can lead to perceived or real self-destruction. Addiction can also lead to perceived or real self-destruction. Our collective addiction to how much we have, such as money; what we do with what we have: the food, the drink and so on; is leading to our self-destruction and that of the planet we live on. Deep down, we know that this is the case. We know if we continue doing what we're doing, there can be only one outcome. But we carry on doing it anyway convincing ourselves the outcome will be different.

That. Is. Insane!

'We drink too much, smoke too much, spend too recklessly, laugh too little, drive too fast, get too angry, stay up too late, get up too tired, read too little, watch TV too much. We have multiplied our possessions, but reduced our values. We talk too much, love too seldom and hate too often. We have learned how to make a living, but not a life. We've added years to life, not life to years.'

George Carlin – American stand-up comedian, actor, author, and social critic

At this point you may be thinking again that I am a revolutionary. Once again, I will reaffirm that I am not. But I know that when we change our mindset we can make the changes necessary for this world and our lives to be brighter, happier, nicer and healthier – for everyone.

My mission is twofold: to change the way we view mental illness, and to change the way the system treats the illness - all for the overall benefit of humanity as a whole, in every way imaginable.

'We cannot solve our problems with the same thinking we used when we created them.'

Albert Einstein – German physicist and founder of the Theory of Relativity

Ever since my seed was planted, I have read everywhere about the stigma surrounding mental health and how it doesn't help this crisis we all face.

This is the definition of 'Stigma':

'A mark of disgrace associated with a particular circumstance, quality or person...'

The Oxford Dictionary

- Does someone proven to be of sound mind, but who has openly and blatantly carried out an act whether it is disgusting or evil, deserve to be stigmatised? If all facts and circumstances are taken into consideration, of course that person should be disgraced.

- Does a human being who is simply suffering from a condition, which the vast majority of the medical profession worldwide views as an illness, deserve the same stigma?

We must realise that it is not a stigma which is preventing change from happening. There is a huge barrier which has been placed around mental illness that is holding back change. So many people simply say; *'It's just them. They need to snap out of it. After all, what have they got to be so sad or angry about? I can do it, so why can't they?'* But is this fair?

The barrier is the fact that we are living in denial. In other words, as the 'I Collective' we simply want to carry on as though we collectively have no real problem and everything is fine to continue as it is, consuming our way to perceived happiness. Well it is not!

The best example of the state of denial we live in, is the way members of our armed forces are treated when they leave the services. Let's take a couple of minutes to ponder this idea.

- The back-breaking, soul-destroying training they endure to be fit enough and ready to fight; fight for their country with the knowledge that they will one day have to kill or be killed; the huge sacrifice they are willing to leave down to chance, a chance which may see them never return home.

- The mental torture of what they have to witness in the heat of battle; then if or when they return home, many of them face a battle which will rage on for the rest of their lives, a battle so fierce that it is all encompassing, a battle so important that at stake is the control of their own mind.

- This is a battle they must win to carry on with their life the way they did prior to joining. Sadly, many do not.

When you consider the fact that these men and women voluntarily put their lives in the hands of their commanders and the enemy for their time in service, you would imagine they would receive all the treatment they may require on returning to civilian life. This could not be further from the truth. The attitude of *'Thank you very much for offering your life for our freedom, good luck in life'* is actually their reality. Or *'Should you ever need any assistance in moving forward after the terror and carnage you have witnessed and been through, please join the back of the queue as would anyone else.'*

How can that be right?

Post Traumatic Stress Disorder has not only torn these men and women apart on leaving active service for their country; in many cases it also tears their family apart leaving many of them jobless, homeless and desperate for the help they wholeheartedly deserve.

While living the way we do in our state of denial, we believe these brave men and women have been through war, so they must be strong enough to get over it and carry on as we all do. That is unfair, unjust and simply wrong. The truth is that they have fought for their country, now their country must have the will to fight for them to be able to live their life as we all do.

'Never give up on someone with mental illness.
When 'I' is replaced be 'We', 'illness' becomes 'wellness.'

Shannon L. Alder – author

If we need any more convincing, let's consider the world we will leave our children and they will live in when we're gone...

Chapter 7:
The debt we owe our children

In this chapter, we will consider the world as our children view it. Anyone with children of any age will relate to what you are about to read. If you are planning to have children in future, you may gain priceless knowledge which will stand you in good stead through your teachings. If you are basking in the glory of having grandchildren, the knowledge you could give them may be priceless. If you do not, sadly cannot, or will not have children, then the knowledge gained may be transferred to those who do.

There is nothing we will not do for our children. If we have little money, we will go hungry ourselves while watching them eat well. We will be uncomfortable in the clothes we wear, to see our children wear their clothes well and look their best. We will sleep restlessly on the floor, while they sleep soundly in the bed we give up for them.

If, on the other hand, we have enough money, then we will provide our children with the best of anything that money will buy proportionately, according to our wealth. That is exactly as it should be and is part of modern human nature. That way, in our minds at least, our children will realise one day – if they do not already – that we, their parents, love them with every molecule of our being.

However, in the natural scheme of things, our children should know that we love them through the love we give, not through the materials we shower them with and the aspirations we have for them. From the moment they are born, our children are exposed to both the good and the bad of the world in which we live. We protect them, from what we perceive to be bad and we highlight all of the good surrounding us. This includes the air we breathe, the water and other goodness we drink, the nutritious food we eat. We try to instill the virtue of being able to sleep well and we educate them in the mechanics of reproduction when the time arrives to discuss the 'birds and the bees'.

We should, at this point in our journey together though, be fully aware of how polluted these functions we perform may have become and the danger that brings for their mind and their body, as well as ours. Remember? We need to realise that to a worrying degree, we are not protecting our children fully from what is bad, due to our perception of good and bad also being polluted or having been turned upside down.

'Treat the Earth well. It was not given to you by your parents,
it was loaned to you by your children.
We do not inherit the Earth from our ancestors,
we borrow it from our children.'

Native American proverb

When I first read that proverb it really stuck with me even though it seemed a little bit upside down to the way I have perceived things. For the purposes of our journey together, let's run with the saying and see where it takes us. Are you ready?

In a nutshell, the above proverb means that everything we do should be for the good of our children and the world that they will continue their journey in when we are gone and then ultimately *'borrow'* from their own children, our grandchildren.

During our children's formative pre-school years, between the ages of one and five, they take in information at an astounding rate. How to eat, crawl, walk, how to talk, and how to behave. Unless they are fed on completely pure food and liquid, they are also exposed to some of the food and drink that they will consume for the rest of their lives. Unfortunately, in the current way of living, they start out on the path, which we – as it is all that we know – think is the best for them in terms of what they eat and drink. On our journey, we have questioned whether, indeed, that is the right path.

If our young children could, they would eat their meals backwards – a main course of cake or pudding and as much of it as possible - followed by a modest dessert of mainly processed meat.

As I write this, I can easily imagine my five-year-old son helping himself to a number of chocolate yogurts for his main course, followed by a small portion of pasta and pesto. He would then treat himself, as a reward for finishing his food, with a couple of chocolate bars. Our job as parents in this instance is to try to limit the amount of sugar our children consume. Is it not? Maybe we could steer them towards a healthier treat of organically grown fruit, juicy and delicious! Do you? Or do you give in to what you know is coming by having the sweet, unhealthy, addictive stuff available? I have been guilty of this in the past: anything for a quieter, more peaceful life, we think as parents! All the while, our children are also taking in what they sense around them, everything that surrounds them. Giving children the toys and other instruments by which they learn all of the functions listed above in these formative years is of crucial importance.

There has to be a healthy balance of bonding, encouragement and help as they enjoy these toys, as well as allowing them to learn and make mistakes for themselves. This is one of the great experiences of parenthood. It can also be one of the most difficult things to cope with as a parent, when the child sets off on one of their monumental, and partially natural, mood swings. Now, this mood swing could simply be down to the fact that they cannot find a small toy they were just playing with and are now sitting on, however, due to the pressures of modern parenthood, which we all go through, sometimes we, understandably may not be able to find the simple answer to our child's woes. So what do we do?

What is the answer to quell this disturbance of the peace when we are too tired and busy to be able to think logically in this din? Sometimes the answer to the above disturbance may be to give them a cuddle and find out exactly what their issue was. If the problem wasn't that they were in need of a meal or drink, or changing their nappy or going for a sleep because it was the right time, then we could engage with them for a short time in finding another game to play. Something that was more fun than the last game, then let them carry on – when happy – on their own. At other times, the quicker answer, in keeping with our daily lives, may be to check that it is not one of their natural needs, remind them that kids television has been on for the whole duration of their tantrum, and get them to sit down watching whatever is on television, while eating and drinking the sugar we have literally given them to maintain the peace. When they get out of their chair, having finished their treat, their renewed energy and enthusiasm can be put down to either contentment, or the rush of the sugar flowing through their veins, until the next tantrum erupts. Although I haven't always, I now know which I'd rather do.

We should follow the commands of our heart in this regard: Turn on the radio for our children rather than the television, make them healthy homemade snacks; including healthy grains, such as granola sweetened naturally with organic honey rather than sugar. If they love crisps, then make them crisps out of organically grown vegetables and fruit. Each of these alternatives would contain most of, if not all of the goodness of the fruit or vegetable, while tasting as sweet if they were naturally sweetened with unprocessed honey. Additionally, they would not give our children anywhere near as much of the chemicals, fats, sugar and additives that the normal treats pollute them with. It's a no-brainer really, isn't it?

When our children say that they do not, or will not eat what is being offered, a battle of wills commences. As parents, we have our will power tested to the very core, but do we give in to their every desire, even though we know it will be bad for their health to restore order or do we stand our ground?

Here's an example from my family life.

Once, after my son came home from school, as usual he enquired what he was having for his dinner. His mother informed him he was going to be eating Shepherd's Pie.

'Ohhh,... But I... I don't like shepherd's pie,' was his reply.

'Well, you've eaten it before, it's very good for you and it will make you big and strong.' Said his mother, calmly and lovingly.

'I don't like it and I am not eating it!' Was our son's assertion. Game on!

Fortunately, the conversation ended there until I got him up to the table in the usual fashion, as his mother was dishing up dinner in the kitchen a few metres away. As he sat at the table, he asked again.

'What are we having for dinner?'

'Shepherd's pie, son.'

He did not reply, but made it very clear he was in a sulk. A few minutes later when we were all sitting at the table, his silence continued as he completely ignored the plate of wholesome homemade food in front of him. So, I tried with some encouragement,

'Son,' I said. 'This shepherd's pie that your mother has made for you is delicious, why don't you try some?'

'I do not like it and I am not eating it!' he shouted.

There was a very short pause before his mother replied before I could.

'I have made you shepherd's pie. If you do not eat it, there will be nothing else for dinner and no dessert.' She said firmly but gently.

We left him with that, continued with our conversation while eating and supervising our daughter's meal, hoping deep down, that our son would also afford us an attempt at his. Within 10 to 15 minutes, our son had finished two helpings of shepherd's pie. After saying how delicious it was, he was waiting for his dessert.

'Mummy, Daddy, I'm full up with shepherd's pie, now can I have my dessert?'

'What's the magic word, son?'

'Please…' He answered, with a beaming smile.

My partner and I both shared a loving, amused glance at one another. That is the way forward, I thought. I think she agreed.

Snow-ploughing towards the edge

In general, when our children start school, they are beginning to learn the skills which they need to acquire to be able to fly from the nest, years later. It is the beginning of one of the most important journeys they will ever make in life.

For example, one day, my son, who had been trying to get my attention for a few seconds before we were about to set off on the school run, shouted.

'Daddy!'

'Yes, sorry, son,' I replied, following my momentary distraction.

'Come on Daddy! I want to go to school and learn!' He enthusiastically demanded.

My pride as we set off for school was only a little smaller in stature than his energetic enthusiasm to set off on his journey.

As we previously agreed, at this point in our journey, we will do anything for our children. This unconditional love extends to helping them to start on their own journey in the best way possible. We all want what's best for our kids, after all they are the future. But what if the way we are helping our children start on their journey of discovery and the way we influence the outcome of that journey is doing more bad than good? Surely that cannot be the case, can it?

We need to realise there are two ends of the scale here.

'A leading education expert says that aggressive parenting makes children; anxious, dependent, narcissistic and careerist.'

The Sunday Times newspaper (Ref. 17)

What is aggressive parenting? Surely we are not aggressive towards our children? Of course, we're not, but this is the top end of the scale. David McCullough, in his book, *You Are Not Special* (Ref. 18) points out that through what he calls, 'snow-plough parenting', children are being nurtured into achievement machines by the blinkered will of their parents clearing the way for them. We can take that argument one step further, in realising that the motivation is the desire to make their children, our children, as likely as possible to be big money earners in this age of consumerism. The stepping-stone towards this goal is high achievement in absolutely everything children do, including going to University.

Do our children view this deep down as conditional love? What do you think?

This approach has led to statistics of one in ten students at British Universities suffering from mental health problems (Ref. 17).

We should understand however, that there could be far more than one in ten due to the state of denial we find ourselves living in. What about those students who are clearly suffering, but putting a brave face on it, not asking to see the doctor? Do they carry on student life well under the mental health radar, hoping not to be disgraced by their underlying struggle to cope? After all, what would their parents, family and friends think if they said they may be suffering from a form of 'mental illness'?

'I've seen my peers sacrifice health, relationships, exploration, activities that can't be quantified and are essential for developing souls and hearts, for grades and cv building.'

William Deresiewicz – American literary critic and author of *Excellent Sheep*

Does this sound familiar to somewhere we've visited on our journey already? Have a think? Perfection, nothing else matters. No one else matters. I must, I must, I must. Who needs quality of life, when you can be at the top of your game and addicted to money, no matter what the cost to your being human?

In other words, we are nurturing our children into results-driven, money-starving perfectionists for whom nothing will ever be good enough to make them truly happy. If they are never happy, you could call that a very simplistic definition of depression. It's a very thin line, isn't it? Surely we do not want to push our children towards being mentally ill by the time they are reaching adulthood and flying the roost towards University? Do we really want that for our children?

Hold on! Where are we parents when all of this is happening?

We parents are out striving to provide the means by which our children can have the very best they can consume depending on what we can afford. Remember? While we are striving at work, they are striving at school. We must not be too critical of the school system here. They do a fantastic job of taking care of our children, day in and day out, during term time, guiding them on their journey of discovery, while we are carrying out our productive role as slaves to money. However, these teachers are not trained as mental health workers. Neither should they be expected to carry out that role. Even if soon they may have to!

At the other end of the scale, I do not condone child cruelty in any way, shape or form. Some hardcore consumers out there may say the assertion of saying no to children when they beg for the treats they desire is unkind or cruel. But is it? Especially when it is for their good health?

Returning to the concept of 'snow-plough' parenting, we need to realise that we have been steered in that direction as a society. For example, one of the most obstructive things we could have ever done for our children here was to allow convention to govern how we as a society are allowed to discipline our children without having clear guidelines on effective discipline. Especially without giving full consideration to the effect it would have on society's children as a whole. In the UK it seems we have almost completely dismantled the means by which we can discipline our children. Could this be a perfect example of what we may perceive to be 'snow-plough parenting'?

Let's take a look. There is a very thin line between discipline and abuse and that line must never be crossed, but it seems we have lacked the courage and conviction to consider and resolutely define where the line is. Our children have suffered hugely as a result. This is where 'snow-plough' parents will believe that what we have done is exactly right.

What have we done?

Firstly, in about 1963, the National Service was abolished in the UK. National Service was another way of saying conscription – the compulsory drafting of young adult men of a certain age – into the Armed Services. It is arguable that the strength of character which this time gave these boys, turned them into fine, upstanding men.

> *'The Army has done amazing things for me. And more importantly to me, what I've seen the Army do for other young guys. You know, I was a Troop Commander in Windsor for three and a half years, but I had eleven guys under my command. And some of these guys were – I mean naughty is not the word – they were on a different level. And their backgrounds and the issues they had. And then over those three years to see the way that they changed is huge.'*

**UK Telegraph Newspaper interview,
His Royal Highness Prince Harry (Ref. 19)**

The article implied that His Royal Highness was calling for the reinstatement of National Service. In this age of professional Armed Services and personal freedom, maybe compulsory National Service is not practical. However, the benefits it brings to those brought under its wing, along with the values of respect, discipline and self-discovery, are priceless. Since 1963, these benefits and values have not been so forcibly instilled in our young men. The freedoms enjoyed by modern society mean that National Service no longer fits. However, the fact that it has not been replaced by another way of instilling those priceless values is what has potentially done harm to our children as a whole.

Secondly, in 1998, corporal punishment was banned by law from UK independent schools. This followed a similar ruling, banning this form of punishment – in the form of a caning – from state schools. As mentioned, the line is too thin between punishment and abuse. Therefore, this move had to be made to protect our children from teachers who may have been viewed as too keen to turn to this form of punishment. However, the fact that we did not replace it with another, effective form of less brutal punishment, is where our children have been let down.

Thirdly, we as parents have become too wary of being seen to discipline our children in too harsh a way. We believe deep down, we will be viewed as acting on the wrong side of the law if we are too harsh on our children in the home or in public. Without clearer guidelines on acceptable child discipline, this is the only logical approach we can take. Especially when we consider the shameful, disgusting, perverse, inhuman and in some cases barbaric situations our Social Services have had to deal with - when children have been killed – yes killed by their so-called guardians.

Our failing, though, has been not to stand together as one and demand direction on what we can and cannot do in disciplining our children. There were two instances in my childhood which illustrate how discipline worked back in my younger days.

On one of my first visits to the beautiful island in the Caribbean where my father was born, my grandfather, another great man, arranged for me to spend a day or a morning at the school where my father started his journey of discovery which saw him take the path towards medicine. From memory, I was around nine or ten at the time of my visit to the school. My memory of the time I spent at the school that day is limited to one thing, one incident, which will always stay with me. The school my father attended had a very good reputation on the island. When you see them making their way to school, the children of the Island are impeccably well-presented from top to toe across the board. This was, and I hope still is, the philosophy of the school system there. You go to school to learn discipline, respect and gain knowledge. You could see these principles shining bright in the way the children looked on their journey to school.

We were herded into a large hall for the school assembly. I do not even have a clear memory of what was said in the assembly because my young ears could not keep up with the use of the English language that I heard. All I remember is a number of boys being taken up on stage by a gentleman, who I imagine was the head teacher or someone of similar standing. In turn each and every one of the boys up on stage was given a hard whack with a slipper on their backside, hard enough to make each and every one of them grimace. They were not hit hard enough for it to be called cruelty, but in my opinion, the very fact they had been made an example of in front of the whole school, served its purpose for them and all the young onlookers. I imagine that anyone foolish enough to behave badly deserved their punishment and would be in line for the same treatment the next day or whenever it was next carried out. Job done.

My father never raised his hand to me nor any of my other siblings; not once. In my mind and from my memory, all he had to do was mention the word belt and I would not only fall straight into line, but also ask how high to jump. Discipline seems to be missing from the lives of our children nowadays. Parents and teachers alike are terrified of the consequences of being labeled as abusers. Excuse the level of generalising at this point, but children of school age are showing all the signs of a complete lack of discipline, respect and caring. Not only for other people around them, whether they are young or old, but also for themselves. Where, generally, is this taking our children?

There have been three incidents in the UK that I can remember from over the last two decades when teachers have been attacked while at or outside a school. Two of these have happened in the last couple of years. They were not attacked by parents no, they have been attacked by children. Two of those teachers died. That's right, they were killed by children of the age that their role was to teach, care for and protect. What is the world coming to when not one teacher but three can be attacked, and in two cases killed, by children? What sort of world – that we have borrowed – are we going to give back to our children? While our children are at school on their journey of discovery, their teachers spend more time with them than we do. These experts in childcare and education are beginning to tell us about the deafening alarm bells they are hearing and the worrying signs they are seeing in our children:

'We've created this epidemic of anxiety for ourselves as a society and if our obligation as educators is to try to the best of our ability to set young people up as best we can for whatever the future may hold, then to ignore this whole area or to trivialise it is really irresponsible.'

Eve Jardine-Young – Headteacher, interviewed by Sky News, 'School May Ban Homework To Combat Depression', June 2015 (Ref. 20)

This quote, for me, sums up the way our children perceive the world they live in. Scary isn't it?

*'Mental health is a massive problem in
Britain in schools and Universities.'*

**Sir Anthony Seldon – Headteacher, interviewed on
Sky News, 'School May Ban Homework To Combat
Depression', June 2015 (Ref. 20)**

*'The World Health Organization in 2014, revealed
that a fifth of 15-year-olds in England said they
had self-harmed in the past twelve months.'*

The UK Telegraph newspaper (Ref. 21)

Again, we have to realise that the figures generated are not the result of the researchers speaking to every 15-year-old in the country. But what about those who have self-harmed and have not admitted it to anyone else?

One journalist expressed her alarm when a teacher at her child's school said that:

*'Probably a third of the year are suffering
from depression, anorexia or self-harming.'*

The UK Telegraph newspaper (Ref. 21)

One in three! Is that not the same statistic as the obesity epidemic we face in years to come? Hold on, this is happening right now! We must remember that these quotes are coming from very intelligent teachers who arguably spend more time with our children than we do. The scariest point, which we must consider is the plight of our children at University.

In the quoted article above, which gives the figure of one in ten students at British Universities suffering from mental health issues, it also states that 50% of 18 year-olds now go to

University. If the World Health Organisation is stating that *a fifth of 15-year-olds in England* were so mentally distressed that they are self-harming, how can their situation have improved by the time they are 18 and at University, when they have been under even more pressure and subjected to even more mental and physical pollution in the mean time? Surely, this means that in reality, at least two in ten University students have mental health problems.

We parents get to see the teachers and find out how our children are doing at school. My child of school age is not old enough yet for his teacher to be having in depth conversations with me about his true progress on his journey, but his enthusiasm fills me with hope. Unfortunately, due to their untrained eye, many teachers may put the concerns they have about any child's bad attitude or behaviour down to the perception that they like to be naughty, but what if these are the very early warning signs of other more serious matters that are being missed at school and at home? What happens then? Nothing!

The battle for the minds of our children

Do you remember when we were considering our response to our child having a tantrum and how to quell the situation? Do you remember that point where the battle of wills starts when we have to say no to our child and mean it? We are finding it almost impossible to stand up to their every request as they grow up, or to limit their exposure to the very things, which are polluting their mind and body. We feel this is the only way we can show our true love for them in the very limited amount of time we get to spend with them as they are growing up. Our attitude has to change. What are the requests or demands our children make as they are growing up?

Do you remember the part of our journey together when we took on board the quote about the industrial revolution happening on a scale of about a second ago?

A famous speech made by British Prime Minister, Harold Wilson called it the *'white heat of technology.'* Using the normal scale of time, that was in 1963, but employing the same scale as in the other quote it was a millisecond ago. Since then we have landed on the moon, invented colour television, computers, internet, smart phones and the hand-held tablet computers, which we can use for anything, from communicating with each other to watching television to listening to music. Through the growth of the age of consumerism and their widespread availability, our children quickly become masters of this technology while we can just about send a text or an email. As with their learning to eat, walk and talk in their formative years, they pick up the use of this technology at an astounding rate. Where is all this technology taking our children, bearing in mind that this has all happened in the past millisecond?

'10 Reasons Why Handheld Devices Should Be Banned for Children Under the Age of 12' is a scary article published by in 2014, by the Huffington Post (Ref. 22) about Steve Jobs, inventor of the iPad, but who did not allow his own children to use them. Why would he do that? We should all be very wary of allowing our children to spend hours and hours playing on or using these devices even though it may give us the solace of some peace and quiet. But why?

Have you ever played a game on one? I have and once you start playing the game, do you not find it extremely difficult to stop and put it down. Imagine the hugely powerful impulses our children experience when playing the same games. The majority of the technology being created, through the way it engages our senses and those of our children even in their formative pre-school years, is also nurturing an addictive side to their nature.

This is another instance where a battle of wills starts with our children but we have to come out on top and limit their use of this technology, for their own sake and for the sake of the world we return to them. We parents, generally speaking, are not winning the battle of wills. We are losing. Why?

My father used to say that the mother is the primary parent. In some senses, he was almost right, but in today's world that simply cannot work in its purest form. We need to understand, quickly, that fathers have as important a role in the rearing of our children. Mothers simply cannot do it all, although they do a great job. However, children desperately need their fathers.

Who else will discipline them - when they are in need of it - at home?

Let's not forget that children need to be constantly shown love and attention by both parents, but when it comes to discipline, there needs to be a bit of good cop bad cop going on. Usually, when it comes to discipline, it is down to fathers to instill discipline and respect into our children's lives. Where are the fathers?

The fathers are either toiling away, day in day out, striving to provide enough money to bring up their children in this era of ever-rising prices and austerity. Or they may have split up with the mother, so they still strive to provide when they do get to see the children, but only have a limited time to repair the broken patchwork, which the children view as the love they once shared as a family. Or they may have completely flown away from the nest which is bringing up their children, viewing their only responsibility as putting money into an account every so often and being content with that, maybe they don't even do that. Or they may be in prison. Or they may, sadly, have passed away. The fact is that wherever we fathers are, we need to do more to help raise our children, while instilling the principles of discipline, respect and caring for ourselves, other people and the world we live in. Unfortunately, we are failing.

Our slavery to money and the fast-paced world we live in, are distracting us to such an extent that we, as parents, are losing the battle of wills badly. In this age of consumerism, life has been turned so much on its head that we view the best way of proving our love for our children is to shower them with all the material possessions that we can afford. But that does not and will not cut it, now or ever. So what will the world be like that we've borrowed from our children, when we inevitably return it to them one day?

Sadly, there is no way of knowing for sure the answer to that question because we cannot see into the future. We can only guess what the world will be like by considering how it is now, as we have in this journey through this book together, and considering how our children are at this point in time.

So, how are our children?

Generally speaking, our children want so much for us to love them in a specific way, but we do not. We love them by giving them all of the things, which we think are great but are in actual fact, damaging their future, so they go with it.

We push them and push them into taking the only path we know, without realising the damage we may be doing to their mental health, so they go with it because they view that as what is expected of them.

We do not discipline them or teach them to care for one another or themselves, so they go with it because we do not show them any other way. Our view of success is instilled as what they should view as success, without any regard for happiness or contentment or loving every inch of the world in which they live. But we show them no other possible version of success, so they go with it. The world that we show them is a virtual one, viewed on a television screen, or computer, or tablet through the world wide web. They get their kicks from rampaging on console games where they get to run havoc and destroy everything in sight. All because we do not have sufficient time to show them the proper love they deserve and instill the virtues they deserve, but they go with it in their own way, online.

As a result, many children have begun exploding into an internal frenzy of violence, where they imagine how they can let off the red hot steam that is the anxiety, panic and depression inside of their minds as a result of the world we are showing them. In some cases, they actually carry out these barbaric acts externally, in the form of killing their teachers – the very people who are helping them start what is supposed to be their wonderful journey of discovery. Or they are killing each other, or, they are killing themselves.

This. Is. What. Is. Happening. Right. Now!

The only way that we can imagine the world of the future is through the eyes of our children. That world which we return to them will be out of control unless change starts happening now. What can we do to make the world we return to our children change, so they can continue that change and hopefully, our grandchildren can begin to reap the rewards of that change and our great grandchildren can blossom? That is the debt which we owe our children.

How are you?

What is your heart saying to you right now?

Are we ready to start making change happen together?

PART THREE:
US

Chapter 8:
The power we have as one

In this chapter, we will remind ourselves of instances where human resolve has turned negative to positive, as in the case of the demise of segregation and apartheid. We will then consider the huge positive effect which unity could have on the current mental health crisis.

Throughout human history, we have blossomed through remarkable feats and achievements. These feats have been achieved when we have come together as one unified force, a very large group of human individuals with a core aim or objective in mind. These may have been ending segregation in America or apartheid in South Africa, but they have had one common characteristic, that a large enough group of human beings came together with a unified set of core aims or objectives and did not stop until those aims or objectives were achieved.

There have been other occasions when a large group of us have unified in such a way as to exploit and unjustly dehumanise another group for no good reason, such as the colour of their skin. When studying what may cause this unjust treatment of humans according to their colour, many conclusions can be drawn. One conclusion is the fear humans have of matters we cannot comprehend. This fear can in some instances be so great that it exists only in our subconscious. The process of fear we go through subconsciously can make us demonise something we do not understand. Alternatively, we may act in denial to such a degree that we can almost convince ourselves it does not exist and that everything will be fine, even though we know deep down that what we are doing is wrong.

The same can be said for mental ill-health to some degree. The lack of comprehension we have about mental health is so great that even the experts in the mental health field cannot pin down the cause of one of the most common forms of mental ill-health present in the modern world – depression and all that it is associated with.

Let's go back to the two examples of South African apartheid and segregation in America. Both regimes were disgusting examples of the type of human behaviour that can prevail when there is a deep-seated sense of misunderstanding in our psyche. The whole world knew that both these regimes were against the very grain of human nature, and the whole world came together in condemning them. However, that was not quite enough, it also took the oppressed in each instance, to stand together in an almost superhuman act of defiance, for each respective regime to disintegrate. The strength of human unity has seen us, as a race, overcome any obstacle that has been in our path.

Possibly one of the greatest obstacles we have ever had to face is right in front of us now. That is the lack of comprehension we have for our own crisis of mental ill health within each and every one of us as a race. The size of this particular obstacle is so great that if we do not overcome it, it could lead to the destruction of us all and our home, Earth.

Why can't we stand together, as one and overcome this obstacle like anything else we have come up against? The simple answer is that we can. However, probably a better question for us to ask ourselves is: Why aren't we standing as one in our battle with mental health?

'This is where we are at right now, as a whole.
No one is left out of the loop. We are experiencing
a reality based on a thin veneer of lies and illusions.
A world where greed is our God and wisdom is sin,
where division is key and unity is fantasy,
where the ego-driven cleverness of the mind is praised,
rather than the intelligence of the heart.'

Bill Hicks – controversial American comedian and social critic

Goal! Try! Touchdown! Six Runs! Home Run! Hole-in-One!

Bill Hicks, more than twenty years ago, hit the nail bang on the head with that one quote, although my interpretation of his words in the world we live in now is somewhat different to his meaning.

Along our journey together in this book, we have made some discoveries. I hope we can all agree that we are in need of change, each and every one of us, as a race of human beings. We are all in the same situation. We can choose to initiate change for the sake of our children, the world we return to them, and for the world they live in, to be able to survive. We do not have to change the way we live in any great way. It is our attitude that needs to change. Once our attitude changes, then other changes will follow on naturally as a result of this change. They will be a bright spark for the whole of humanity, our individual or collective health and ultimately the health of our home, Earth, which we will one day return to our children.

We have discovered during our journey, that we have erected a barrier of denial to protect the lack of comprehension we have about our own mental health. The state of denial in which we live represents the 'reality based on a thin veneer of lies and illusions' as Hicks put it. That barrier has allowed us to continue on our greedy, blinkered quest as an ego-driven 'I Collective', on our selfish, self-destructive pursuit of money and all that it helps us to consume. We have become so blinkered in this pursuit we have completely forgotten about the virtues with which we have conquered every other obstacle we have come up against before in our brief history. These are the virtues of '…wisdom… unity' and '…the intelligence of the heart.'

What is your heart saying to you right now?

As a collective, the wisdom we need to rediscover is the power we have as one. This power has seen us evolve from the first humans at the middle to lower end of the food chain, to being the kings and queens of our home, the Earth. The intelligence of the heart, which we exhibit in coming together to climb the, until now, insurmountable obstacle of our own mental health, is unity. Unity in every sense of the word – our attitude, diagnosis, treatment, ongoing recovery, social and economic empowerment through constructive empathy – will help us get over this obstacle. This will ultimately result in a system where all the human resources and components work in unity.

We hear everywhere that it is very important to talk and have conversations about mental health. Not only is talking therapeutic, but it raises awareness of the seriousness of our mental health crisis. If the message conveyed in this book formed the basis of the widespread conversation about mental health, then change will have already started to happen.

Chapter 9:
The Conception of Unity

In this chapter, we will explore the meaning of Unity Conception, prior to applying this meaning to the overall mental health crisis. When we look up the definition of unity, there are certain words and phrases that stand out.

'...the state or quality of being one; oneness.
The act, state, or quality of forming a whole from separate
parts; uniformity or constancy...'

The Oxford Dictionary

Looking up the definition of conception, the same can be said.

'...something conceived; notion, idea, design or plan;
origin or beginning...'

The Oxford Dictionary

Remember there are two concerns for us:

1. to change the way we view mental illness; and

2. to change the way the system treats the illness.

The unity we need to show, relates to these two areas.

Firstly, we have to change our perception of mental illness while realising that to a certain extent, it is in each and every one of us. This is not a suggestion that each and every one of us is mentally ill. It is the way that we are operating as a society, which is making us individually more susceptible to mental illness. The stigma or state of denial in which we live, reinforces this susceptibility.

As the World Health Organisation stated in 2001, 15 years ago, 450 million people suffered from some form of mental illness. Around 350 million people worldwide suffer from depression alone. What about all the other disorders, which are included in the mental health umbrella? The number of people suffering in silence who are too afraid of the disgrace of getting a diagnosis? And worryingly, what about the number of children affected? Reportedly, children as young as ten require help for suicidal thoughts according to The Sun Newspaper (Ref. 23). The current figure could be more than a billion people of all ages suffering worldwide. Let's consider the fact that all these people have families and friends who have to witness – while not fully understanding – the illness of their friend or loved one. This could mean that every single person on the planet is touched first or second hand, by mental health without even knowing it.

Without a change of attitude, we will carry on along the same path. Unless we realise this and change the way we view our collective state of mind, then more and more of us, including our children, may become more vulnerable to mental ill health. More and more of us could become what we define as being mentally ill. This includes our children showing the same early signs of vulnerability. This change of attitude will lead to us viewing mental health with constructive empathy rather than outright denial or disgrace. By supporting these views, talking about them openly and doing the same for the overall vision to follow, you will have changed your attitude. By encouraging other people to take the same journey we are currently on, you will have hopefully set them off on the same journey. Everyone who makes this journey should reach the destination of unity, forming a whole new group attitude with the same core belief which originally set me off on my journey: the core belief that the whole realm of mental ill health has to change.

Once that core belief is held by enough individuals around the world, forming a whole in terms of their new-born attitude, the oneness which will prevail will allow uniformity and constancy in the way we as a society view mental ill health and also health in the way, which we as a whole are living, will come to the fore. Nowadays, the possibility of as many people as humanly possible upholding this attitude is easy, due to modern technology, which is available to us all in one form or another. Almost all of the information, which we have noticed, has started opening our eyes about what we are doing to ourselves and to our world is available at the touch of a few buttons. The vast majority of this information is open for all to see and has been taken from various sites through their presence on social media.

We have become more interconnected as a race of human beings than ever before. We now must make it work for us, for the good of our collective mental health, by spreading the word to every corner of the world in which we live, all through clicking a few buttons and spreading the unity we can find in ourselves, individually, and coming together to form one collective attitude towards the barrier that we will overcome together.

Secondly, we should wholeheartedly believe that almost everything that needs to be in place for the effective 'cradle to grave to cradle' treatment required in this mental health crisis we face, already exists. I can only speak for the case in the UK, because that is what I have seen and experienced second hand from my family members. I have not received the treatment, but I have seen the treatment that is given to those suffering, while their loved ones have to sit in silence and bite their tongues.

The vision that follows is taken from what I have observed as being the case in this country. Almost everything required for effective treatment already exists. The huge problem we have and what causes the system here to fail so miserably, is the fact that it does not operate as a whole made up of separate parts, mainly due to a woeful lack of investment. All the individual parts act as their own whole and none of the individual parts, which make up the so-called system, know what any of the other individual parts are doing. When dealing with a crisis, this is not the way to break it down, this is the way to make the crisis even worse. The separate parts of this system need to be brought together in unity and combined to make one, well-oiled, efficient machine with the core objective of meeting this crisis head on and overcoming it.

The conception phase of the solution for this crisis originated with the seed that was planted within me by the commands of my heart. It was planted as a result of the promise I made to my father when I said goodbye to him and the desperate circumstances which have unraveled ever since. The conception we have been through together on our journey has led to the impending birth of Unity. This conception will make it possible for me and those surrounding me to free the cogs of the machine which our newfound attitude will form part of, and make the vision you are about to imagine, as clear as a rainbow in our reality, when the sun is beaming after a storm.

That is the most important promise I need to make to you - the reader - and absolutely everyone who takes this journey. Please ponder for a moment.

What can we do to overcome the mental health crisis threatening our being?

If you have any thoughts or suggestions, please do not hesitate to get in touch: progress@unity-mhs.org

Chapter 10:
The Unity Vision

We in Unity will never judge the individual. Our only concern is to promote quick, efficient and ongoing treatment for those in need with a view to creating a positive individual, social and economic impact throughout the UK and wherever necessary throughout the World.

In 1948, the National Health Service was born in the UK. It was groundbreaking. At the heart of its conception was the pillar of providing universal treatment, free at the point of delivery, for legal residents of the UK. At the time and since then, it was viewed as a shining example of how the state should provide health care for those individuals who together make the state whole. That is what drew my father here in the 1960s to practice in the profession which he would one day excel in. However, times have changed. At the time of its birth, the National Health Service was built on principles and mechanics for it to be able to cater for the population of the UK, a population, which in 1948, was approximately 50 million people. Between 1948 and 2005, that population increased by around 10 million.

'The office for National Statistics in the UK has projected that the population will increase by another 10 million in the next 15 years if the current trends continues.'

BBC News Channel Online (Ref. 24)

The National Health Service is beginning to develop very big cracks, as it begins to wilt under the pressure of this population growth.

Additionally, in 1948 when the service was born, mental health was, rightly or wrongly, not viewed as the problem that it is today. Over the past decades, treatment has moved from institutional asylum treatment for mental illness towards community care, where sufferers can work through their recovery:

'Its [community care] main goal is to empower and emancipate people with psychiatric and social problems, enabling them to be fully participating members of society.'

The Mental Health Foundation (Ref. 25)

This is the theory of best practice used by the modern world or the majority of it. If this is the route to take then, on paper at least, it works. However, it is how this treatment works in practice that should be our main concern.

How is this mode of treatment working in practice?

We believe there is a huge gap in mental health treatment between the NHS & the private sector. The families of those suffering are stuck in the middle not knowing which way to turn.

The NHS is universally free at the point of delivery, but the waiting times involved due to the immense pressure it is under, make it virtually undeliverable for the effective treatment of mental health issues.

By their very nature, mental health problems are unique. It is the only area of health where the patient may not realise they are ill because they do not notice the symptoms, or even accept the fact that they are ill once diagnosed. Therefore, we believe that effective treatment has to be instantly available at a very specific point in time. This is when the sufferer holds up their hands and declares *'I am ill and I need help!'* As a result, the waiting time of weeks or more, often months, for effective treatment under the already over-stretched NHS renders it undeliverable when it is most needed. During those few moments when the sufferer makes their declaration, then and only then during their brief time of clarity, they are not potentially a threat to themselves.

On the other hand, there is the treatment available through the private sector. There are limited spaces available in private residential mental health treatment centres throughout the country. The treatment through these privately run facilities is arguably available quicker than through the NHS. However, the cost of treatment for the sufferer and their family amounts to thousands of pounds per week. The treatment needed is sadly out of reach for the vast majority of those who need it throughout the country. In a limited number of cases, where private treatment may potentially be funded by the local authority, the waiting time issue arises again.

We must believe that when dealing with complex mental health, even one week can be too long, and allows the possibility of the sufferer coming to harm when the illness reduces their mental capacity to battle the demons within. It is logical that early detection is crucial in the treatment of mental health issues. Given the nature of mental health and the fact that in most cases of mental ill health, the sufferer will fight tooth and nail to prove, as they believe, that they are perfectly sound, how is early detection possible?

We must believe that it is only possible through the observance of the family and friends of the person who may be suffering. This is daunting as it is arguable that one of the common and unfortunate side effects of a mental health issue is for the sufferer to alienate themselves or be alienated by their family and friends. The only people who can potentially make them understand there is an issue at hand, unless they realise it themselves, before it is too late. Therefore, throughout the UK there needs to be widespread public education relating to how various mental health issues manifest themselves and the related symptoms they cause. Then and only then, will early detection become possible.

How many families do you know who have had to cope with mental health issues? Each and every one of those families needs to become one in Unity.

Although some of our current number may have worked in healthcare and lend their knowledge, none of us currently practice in healthcare. What we all share is the passion to facilitate change and try to prevent other people from going through the frustration and pain of the disjointed treatment that sufferers receive. Instead, through Unity, we must promote, facilitate and co-ordinate instant effective treatment of mental health issues. Our vision is to make it happen by actively bridging the gap between the NHS and private sector treatment and ultimately making this treatment available universally.

We are calling for all the family and all the friends of all those who have suffered or are suffering from mental health issues to come together in unity, in a bid to bridge this gap. With strength in numbers worldwide, we can make the core belief that we share as near to reality as possible. With that strength in unity, our ultimate vision is to make instant universal mental health treatment available under the same principles at the core of the NHS. In line with this treatment, in the UK there are now countless social enterprises whose vision it is to empower people who are recovering from mental health issues. We will seek to promote, facilitate and coordinate the services which these enterprises offer, with a view to reducing the current reliance and pressure on the: NHS, police and welfare, all of which cost the economy well in excess of 100 billion pounds every year! Instead we want to create a positive social impact and a positive economic impact, by getting those in a certain position back to work and if necessary into social housing. We believe that treatment should never end before time, neither should individual, social and economic empowerment.

What benefits do you imagine could blossom if such changes were to take place first in the UK and then spread to other countries throughout the world, where similar change is needed? Please feel free to let us know your thoughts: www.unity-mhs.org/contact-us

Chapter 11:
The figures do not add up!

At this point, let's for a minute or two, reminisce about a much earlier part of our journey together. Do you remember the inventor who designed a way of cleaning our seas? We considered the number of problems that his invention could potentially solve concerning the water shortage, deadly drinking water and rising sea levels, altogether at the same time. My possible over-excitement about his invention and the possibilities it opens up for the human race, may have been a bit over simplistic and ill conceived, but there was a thought process full of my possibly misplaced imagination.

That style of thinking could be called multi-level problem solving. Sound cool? Why don't you give it a go? Let's use another couple of related examples.

Recently, France made it illegal for supermarkets to bin tons and tons of 'out of date' food every day. Instead, these large organisations will have to give this surplus food to charity. Brilliant, that is a great idea. What about on a global scale? Food Tank published some very interesting facts in an article called *10 facts you might not know about food waste* (Ref. 26, as follow:

> *'1.3 billion tons of food are wasted every year.'*

Wow! Really?

'Just one quarter of all wasted food could feed the 795 million undernourished people around the world who suffer from hunger.'

How many?! What? Really?

'Food waste generates 3.3billion tons of carbon dioxide, which accelerates global climate change.'

Have a think about these three facts for one minute and see what you come up with.

Firstly, a quarter of the food which we waste globally could feed all of those people who are, in some cases, starving to death globally. Surely, the reason why they are not getting this wasted food is that we are worried it will be inedible by the time it reaches those in need? In that case, ship it to them in refrigerated containers as soon as it is deemed unwanted by the primary consumer, those of us who bought the food in the first place. Some of the food – let's say three quarters of it, for argument's sake – is so perishable it would not last that journey: namely, the fruit and vegetables. So what could we do?

Secondly, excuse me again if my answer here is overly simplistic, but once again, humour me because there is a valid point. The problem we face with the lands that have been ravaged by drought is that they have become infertile. It may be very difficult to grow any crops on it. Those crops also need water to flourish.

Let's try this for an idea.

The perishable food such as fruit and vegetables could be used in two ways. One, it could be broken down into compost on a huge scale. That compost could be, in some way, added to this infertile land to make it more fertile and more likely to yield the crops needed by those who are still undernourished today, in the world of the 21st century.

Two, the seeds from some of these fruit and vegetables could be used to conceive new crops or reintroduce old ones that have all but disappeared due to drought. However, if it's not going to rain, nothing will grow. What about the drought? If water will not come to the land, bring water to it. If the water that our friend the 'sea-cleaner' purified, could be used to feed the land and help these crops grow. Additionally, we could use the water being produced by the ice caps, which are melting?

Three, by using the thrown away food we waste each year in this constructive way, we would stop, or at the very least reduce, the three billion tons of carbon dioxide, which this food waste produces.

Could this set of ideas work?

What do we think?

It could, maybe, possibly be workable or maybe it isn't, but this is the way that we, as a race, need to start thinking for our own sake, for the sake of our children and the sake of the planet we live on.

Now, let's look at the mental health crisis we face in the same way. Once again, we will have to use the UK as our base for these thoughts, so if you are not in the UK while taking this journey, please imagine you are here.

Since the credit crunch of 2008, like many other countries around the world, the UK has been seeking a way of reducing its debt, which it relies on to function economically. As a result of the banking crisis, which followed the credit crunch, this was deemed by the government to be crucial. The fact that Greece – a very proud nation – was literally teetering on the edge and very, very close to becoming bankrupt, is the greatest example of why drastic economic action was deemed necessary, and rightly so in one way or another. The solution, which has been employed, is called austerity. On the face of it, these are desperate measures for desperate times. Basically, the government has committed to cut its spending across the board. The theory behind this is that if the government is not spending as much money, it will not have to borrow as much money and increase the UK's debt level. Additionally, the UK Government wants to pay back the majority of the debt we owe as a state, so it can run the country without incurring debt.

That's the way I understand it anyway. This means the cuts in spending being made are particularly severe, affecting all areas of public services, including welfare payments to low earners and those living in poverty; less money being available to pay for policing, and health care.

'Some of the care that is received by people in a moment of crisis in mental health is frankly unacceptable. It is a National scandal.'

Norman Lamb – former Minister of State for Care and Support

It is worth us realising at this point, that the health care provided in times of personal crisis was as scandalous prior to the credit banking crises. Mental health is not high on the list of priorities for the NHS and it never has been. How can there be any possible improvement to the care being offered for what the government acknowledges as a mental health crisis, when all of the cuts being made in NHS funding will be felt most by those sections of the NHS not deemed as high priority, such as mental health? There will be no improvement. In fact, it could be argued that the quality of care will fall even lower. However, the country as a whole will be all right because it is reducing its debt by not spending as much. Value for money has become a big factor in the quality of care afforded to its citizens and those holding the status of being legal residents in the UK. Debt or no debt, how can that be right?

There has been a campaign revolving around the supposed fact that one in four people in the UK suffer from mental health issues. That means that – going by approximate population figures – there are approximately 15 million people in the UK suffering from mental ill health. Additionally, in theory, that means every single person in the UK knows someone who is suffering from these mental health issues. Taking into consideration the number who fall through the cracks, that means the realistic figure could be one in three or even one in two. It is alarming that mental health seems not to be considered a priority then, isn't it?

'UK Government statistics show 46% of people receiving £101 a week Employment and Support Allowance have mental health issues, meaning that new rules could apply to 260,000 people.'

The Huffington Post, 2014 (Ref. 27)

Employment and Support Allowance is a benefit payment made to people in this country who are unable to work due to illness. In their somewhat misplaced wisdom, the Government have come up with the idea of starting to cut the payments made to people who suffer from mental illness.

They plan to do this by making them get some form of therapy, which is deemed good enough to help them back to work. What they fail to realise is that the stress this causes the sufferers and the pressure it puts them under is likely to cause their condition to worsen. Where is the sense in that? Why is the Government taking this stance?

When considering the rolling out of this potential policy, the Government has looked at the situation with only one thing in mind; money. I assume their calculation in this matter would be something along the lines of; *'260,000 people receive £101 per week. So every week, the Department for Work and Pensions (DWP) is paying out more than £26 million. That adds up to £1.365 billion per year.'*

If we could hear the conversations behind closed doors, the Government's attitude to this amount of money being paid out may be something along the lines of: *'It's them. They need to snap out of it. After all, what have they got to be so sad or angry about? Anyway, we cannot afford to be paying them that much every week, month or year. We have huge debts to pay off. They simply have to get on with it and get back into work like everyone else!'*

Does this attitude sound familiar?

The tool, which the State use to determine whether someone is eligible for Employment and Support Allowance is called a Work Capability Assessment (WCA). The way these assessments are carried out and the results they produce have been the subject of growing criticism.

'There is now a significant body of evidence that the WCA is failing to assess people's fitness for work accurately and appropriately, with people who are seriously physically and

mentally ill being found fit for work and those with acute, transient episodes being assessed as lacking capacity and treated in the same way as those with a longer-term prognosis.

Appeals against the decisions are running at approximately 50% and around half of those appeals are upheld. The cost to the taxpayer from this alone is £50m, with a similar amount being spent on reassessment. The DWP is now under significant pressure to publish data on the number of people who have died whilst claiming out-of-work disability benefits.'

Professor Jamie Hacker Hughes – Former President of the British Psychological Society (Ref. 28)

We should compare them to making someone who has never even been into a swimming pool - let alone learnt to swim - jump into the deep end of a swimming pool and search around on the bottom of the pool for several gold coins.

It's just not going to work is it? It could even do them more harm than good. There's no sense in it is there? The figures that the Government is using do not add up.

Let's have a go at it ourselves and see what we can come up with by applying some simple logic to the situation. Before we do though, there's something we have to bear in mind.

One of the big pillars of current UK Government policy is their determination to make £12 billion worth of cuts to the amount being paid in benefits. That figure dwarfs the amount they plan to cut in Employment and Support Allowance (ESA) payments and shows how truly harsh life will become for those already living on the thin line between existence and poverty.

Ready, right, let's go!

Carrying out a simple search on the internet for 'national cost of mental health treatment UK' provides the following quote.

'In England alone, mental illness costs more than £105.2 billion a year, through the cost of medical or social care, production output losses and a monetary valuation of the intangible human cost of disability, suffering and distress. In Scotland, the total cost of mental illness is £8.6 billion, which is equivalent to about 9% of its GDP; in Northern Ireland the cost is £2.8 billion and in Wales £7.2 billion a year.'

The Mental Health Foundation (Ref. 29)

How did you read the above?

To me it says, that across the UK, the total cost of mental health is £123.8 billion. If those figures do not include the amount paid out in benefits for support and housing to those suffering from mental ill health, then that figure will be significantly greater. Regardless of what is included, that dwarfs the amount of cuts that the Government aims to make to the welfare bill. Unfortunately, we cannot be certain whether all of the true extra costs related to mental illness are taken into consideration by the research on the economic burden above. Assuming they are not, let's raise a few questions at this point.

- What is the cost of policing related to mental health, considering that a significant amount of crime may be in some way related to undiagnosed mental illness, while cuts are being made to the policing budget?

- What is the cost of imprisoning people who have

committed a crime, but not been diagnosed as mentally ill, which they may well be?

- What if, as in so many cases that we have been through already, a lot of our problems can be solved and the solution is staring us right in the face?

- What if we were not only able to treat mental illness, but also try to prevent it from happening in the first place?

- What if we could turn all of the negatives that we face into positives?

- What would the multi-level benefits be for us, the country, or the world?

- How would our children benefit?

The figures which the Government obsesses about are not working, and the answer to a great deal of our problems is staring us straight in the face, while we look with thinly veiled pity at those who are suffering from mental illness in silence.

If the people suffering from mental illness were cared for in a proper manner so they could cope with their illness, they would be able to live a free life again. If, once they were showing signs of sustained recovery and at the same time re-training, they could start to work again free from receiving the benefits, which make them feel useless. Instead they could feel they are finally worth something and that life is worth living again. If they were working, they would be making a valuable contribution to the economy through the amount they generate in monetary production and taxes, which would make the amount of cuts the Government wants to make look like a drop in the ocean. If they were well and not having to go in and out of police cells and hospital wards, where is the cost to the police or NHS? A negative would have truly become a positive in every possible sense.

Would such overwhelming austerity be a necessity?

I don't think so, do you?

All that's really necessary for this to happen, is overcoming the obstacle of mental ill health in a logical, well-rounded comprehensive way in all aspects from prevention, early diagnosis, and care, to re-employment, while showing constructive empathy to the plight of those suffering. And also preventing it from happening in the first place, by being mindful of the way we live with our new found attitude.

That's it!

Someone who is suffering from mental illness is made to realise they need help and accept the help on offer; they are lead in a conscientious way through their treatment, while rebuilding their life in every way. They are helped to retrain in a field of choices they are given, only when the time and their improved condition is right. If necessary they are re-housed. They get back into work and are helped, in every way possible, to regain the self-esteem they have desired for so long. They carry on living life in happiness, free of the shackles within their mind.

What if all the work that this new, revitalised, re-energised work force, filled to the brim with enthusiasm, did, was aimed towards the benefit of our health and that of our planet? We will have taken the first step together in making the world, which we will one day return to our children, a safer, brighter, happier and healthier place.

This is what will happen through the Unity of attitude we have formed together on this journey. That is my promise to you, the reader, and absolutely everyone who takes this journey. With the spirit of your support behind us in combination with the strength it gives us, we will make it happen by harnessing the expertise all of the groups and bodies already in existence and, where necessary, creating new groups to fill the gaps required.

Although talking about things is great and must be done to help this change in attitude spread worldwide, it is also high time we stopped only talking about the crisis in mental health we face as the human race, and make things happen for the good of us all.

How do we aim to make this happen with the vision we have?

Chapter 12:
How?

In this chapter, we examine why there may be such a woeful level of investment in mental health care in the UK. It is not viewed as a vote winner. This leads us onto details about how Unity will seek to reverse this trend, by creating a huge community of like-minded individuals with the core belief that the UK will become a world leader in mental health care, once the Unity vision is accepted into the mainstream approach to care.

The simmering mental health crisis in the UK alone is huge. Let's put it into context through a quick and simple calculation. Again, excuse me if this is somewhat over-simplified, but the context here is important.

There are currently around 13 million people suffering from some form of mental illness in this country, which has a total population of 64 million people.

If each of these 13 million people has three family members, it equates to an extra 39 million people affected directly or indirectly, whether they know it or not.

If you add into this scenario that the 13 million sufferers have at least one very close friend, that adds a further 13 million people affected directly or indirectly.

So, theoretically, 13 million sufferers, plus 39 million family members, plus 13 million close friends of sufferers, adds up to 65 million. That is more than the current population of the UK.

Using this simple calculation, it is strongly arguable that whether we are aware of the suffering or not, every single person in this country is affected by mental health directly, indirectly, in one-way or another. Also, it is arguable that mental health will not be given the same importance as physical health until there is a wholesale shift in attitude away from the shame and embarrassment, towards compassion for those suffering from mental ill health.

This book is the seed from which that shift should grow.

It is sad that there is a strong argument that a small majority of the political parties do not view mental health as a vote winner. If they did, surely there would be greater true investment in services rather than the tragic cuts. The truth of the matter is that we can make mental health into a vote winner. Yes, we can. This is where Unity Mental Health Service (MHS) comes in.

How can Unity MHS make this happen?

Unity MHS is a not-for-profit company limited by guarantee, which means there are no shareholders. It takes this legal form so its core motivation is to make the Unity vision - described earlier on in our journey together - a reality. Any profit will form the foundations of sustainability through re-investment.

If the message portrayed in this book can reach every corner of the country, then a huge step will have been taken towards challenging the way society views mental health. Word-of-mouth is the key in challenging perceptions of the crisis.

As a community movement, Unity MHS will go through various stages of development.

1. Unity is bringing people together from all walks of life throughout the UK – giving as much or even as little as they can each month – to tackle the mental health crisis as a community movement in the form of people-powered mental health care. This community has the Unity vision as its driving force along with openness and accountability on the part of the company.

2. This community will mobilise a wide range of resources including knowledge of suffering, compassion, expertise in the field, word-of-mouth and harness the energy, which the student population – being future leaders – will generate with their input. The financial resources generated by this community will be channeled towards helping under-funded private centres to continue their work, the foundations for new (in and outpatient) mental health centres to be secured nationwide, and other related projects which Unity aims to undertake.

3. The growing community will spread the vision while producing further solutions through the knowledge pool and inspired imagination generated throughout its numbers. Most importantly, the financial and other resources available will allow these self-sustaining plans to be built on in the medium term. The momentum that the movement generates will mean the results of our revolutionary approach will become glaringly apparent.

4. With the strength of public support, results in terms of effective ongoing treatment and positive socio-economic results behind it, Unity will have truly made effective

mental health care a vote winner. Once the organisation forms part of the State mechanics - as part of the NHS or a separate department working alongside the NHS - then long may it continue with the assurance that the Unity vision and core values remain front and centre.

Now, before we all set off to spread the word, there are a few questions to ponder. They all relate to parts of what Unity MHS is setting out to achieve.

- If future generations learn at a young age that it is wrong for people who suffer from mental ill health to be ashamed or embarrassed for any reason, would mental health continue to be linked with shame and embarrassment?

- If primary, secondary and senior schools took a proactive approach to minimising stress, if they spot the possible early signs of mental distress in their pupils, and if there was a system in place that prevented them from falling through the net, what would be the positive effects of early intervention in mental health care for the future of those who may be suffering, and for the burden placed on the NHS?

- If those in higher education and at University in the UK were invited to shape the future of mental health policy, with their best ideas being actively put into practice, how much could that improve the lives of millions of people in this country and possibly worldwide, now and in the future?

- If people suffering from mental ill health were given the compassionate care, up to and beyond the point where they could be socially and economically active, proportionate to their ability to do so, how huge would the impact be socially and economically?

Unity MHS is beginning to form partnerships with the wide range of services here in the UK who try to improve lives.

What can you do to drive this movement forwards to make this country a world leader in mental health care?

Chapter 13:
Spread the word

To finish, what can you, the reader, do to end the so-called stigma surrounding mental health and make the UK a world leader in mental health care?

From Thomas Edison's light bulb and Henry Ford's V8 engine, to Timothy Berners-Lee creating the world wide web, we truly have created miracles in recent times. All these miracles have started out as a single, solitary thought fed and grown by imagination. That thought has evolved into a plan. That plan has been put into action, backed by the desire to make it happen no matter what obstacles arise. Nothing is impossible.

Unity is the representation of the thought that I had. My plan, in one sentence, is to make the UK a world leader in the field of mental health care and socio-economic empowerment for sufferers. Absolutely no obstacle will stop that from happening. Unity MHS is the embodiment of my plan being put into action. In comparison to the miracles noted above, our task is relatively simple because the foundations already exist for the care in this country to be unrivalled. They simply need to be harnessed and led in the correct direction as one, united effort.

With your support and the support of enough of the population that is exactly what we will do. The results for those in need of care will be astounding. The social and economic impact will be breath taking. All of this will be created by your decision to tell everyone you know about joining the Unity community.

Following the journey, which we have started on together, through this book and now through your word-of-mouth, we can create the positive, 'can do' attitude we need to make change happen.

'So powerful is the light of unity, that it can illuminate the whole Earth.'

Bahaullah –Tehraniain propher and founder of the Bahai Faith

Thank you very much in advance, for spreading the word. Hopefully you will be part of a movement which will improve millions of lives now and ever onwards.

Please join our mailing list and help spread the word far and wide.

www.unity-mhs.org

References and Further Reading

The majority of the quotes in this book are from social media sources, as below. For website addresses of articles, please see Research page on www.unity-mhs.org

Chapter 2: Whose suffering serves as inspiration?

1. Bedell, Geraldine. (27th February 2016) 'Teenage mental health crisis: rates of depression have soared in the past 25 years', *The Independent newspaper website.*

Chapter 4: Where have I been and what have I learnt?

2. Schocker, Laura. (15th August 2015) '16 Super Successful Introverts', *The Huffington Post website.*

3. Watkins, Light. (20th May, 2015) 'Seven surefire signs you're following your heart.' www.mindbodygreen.com

4. The World Health Organisation (2001). 'Mental disorders affect one in four people'.

Chapter 5: Who are we?

5. Carrington, Damian. (13th June 2016) 'Air pollution linked to increased mental illness in children,' *The Guardian newspaper website.*

6. The USGS Water Science School website: https://water.usgs.gov/edu/earthhowmuch.html

7. Helmenstine, Anne Marie PhD, scientist. (March 2017). https://www.thoughtco.com/how-much-of-your-body-is-water-609406

8. United Nations, World Water Day 2103: http://www.unwater.org/water-cooperation-2013/water-cooperation/facts-and-figures/en/

9. Griffiths, Sarah. (9th September 2013) 'Could a teenager save the world's oceans? Student, 19, claims his invention could clean up the seas in just five years', *The Dail Mail newspaper website*

10. The American Heart Association: http://www.heart.org

11. Smith, Rebecca. (17th October 2007) 'Half of adults will be obese by 2050', *The Telegraph newspaper online*

12. *Fed Up. It's Time to Get Real About Food*; a film by Stephanie Soechtig: http://fedupmovie.com

13. Podcast; Tim Stoddart, (30th June 2015); on the Sober Nation website: http://www.sobernation.com/what-do-drugs-and-sugar-have-in-common/

14. Enders, Giulia. *Gut: The Inside Story of Our Body's Most Underrated Organ* (2015, Scribe UK)

15. Mercola, Dr. (29th June 2015) 'The surprising root cause of anxiety and depression', *Waking Times website*

16. *The Matrix*, 1999, a science fiction film written and directed by The Wachowski Brothers

Chapter 7: The debt we owe our children

17. Griffiths, Sian. (24th August 2014) "Snowplough' parents can ruin children's lives', *The Sunday Times newspaper website*

18. McCullough, David. *You Are Not Special* (2015, Ecco Press)

19. Harley, Nicola. (16th May 2015) 'Prince Harry calls to bring back National Service', *The Telegraph newspaper website*

20. 'School may ban homework to combat depression' (6th June 2015), *Sky News website*

21. Pearson, Allison. (6th June 2015) 'A*s in fear, misery and self-harm', *The Telegraph newspaper website*

22. Rowan, Cris. (3rd June 2014) '10 Reasons Why Handheld Devices Should Be Banned for Children Under the Age of 12', *The Huffington Post website*

Chapter 9: The Conception of Unity

23. Lockett, Jon. (8th September 2016) 'Kids as young as 10 are now considering suicide as calls to Childline doubles in five years', *The Sun newspaper website*

Chapter 10: The Unity vision

24. 'UK population to rise "to rise by 71.6m" (21st October 2009), *BBC News website*

25. Baudin, D., McCulloch, A., Liegweois, A. *Brief History of Specialist Mental Health Care*, (2002, The Mental Health Foundation)

Chapter 11: The figures do not add up!

26. *'10 Facts You Might Not Know About Food Waste', Food Tank website*: https://foodtank.com/news/2015/06/world-environment-day-10-facts-about-food-waste-from-bcfn/

27. Elgot, Jessica. (13th July 2014) 'Tories Plan To Make Mental Health ESA Claimants Prove They Are Really Depressed', *Huffington Post website*

28. Hacker-Hughes, Prof. Jamie. (9th June 2015) 'Welcome for our call of the Work Capability Assessment', *The British Psychological Society website*

29. The Mental Health Foundation, in association with King's College London, *'Economic burden of mental illness cannot be tackled without research investment'* (2010)